Treatment of Dysphagia in Adults

Resources and Protocols in English and Spanish

Treatment of Dysphagia in Adults
Resources and Protocols in English and Spanish

Maria Provencio-Arambula, M.A.
Dora Provencio, M.A.
M. N. Hegde, Ph.D.

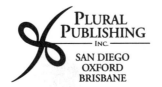

PLURAL PUBLISHING INC.
SAN DIEGO
OXFORD
BRISBANE

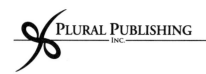

PLURAL PUBLISHING
INC.

5521 Ruffin Road
San Diego, CA 92123

e-mail: info@pluralpublishing.com
Web site: http://www.pluralpublishing.com

49 Bath Street
Abingdon, Oxfordshire OX14 1EA
United Kingdom

Library of Congress Cataloging-in-Publication Data:

Provencio-Arambula, Maria.
    Treatment of dysphagia in adults : resources & protocols in English
and Spanish / Maria Provencio-Arambula, Dora Provencio, M.N.
Hegde.
        p. ; cm.
    Includes bibliographical references and index.
    ISBN-13: 978-1-59756-096-2 (softcover)
    ISBN-10: 1-59756-096-0 (softcover)
    1. Deglutition disorders--Treatment.   I. Provencio, Dora.
II. Hegde, M. N. (Mahabalagiri N.), 1941-   . III. Title.
    [DNLM: 1. Deglutition Disorders--therapy. 2. Adult. 3. Clinical
Protocols. 4. Speech Disorders--therapy.   WI 250 P969t 2007]
RC815.2.T742 2007
616.3'2306--dc22

                                                        2006023291

Contents

Preface

The *Webster's II New College Dictionary* defines a protocol as "a plan for a scientific experiment or treatment." An effective plan for treatment needs to be as clear and precise as a scientific experiment. The concept of protocols, therefore, is eminently suitable for treatment of swallowing disorders in adults.

Treatment in swallowing disorders is primarily a matter of carefully and expertly managing a complex interaction between neurophysiological factors and a chain of learned as well as reflexive behaviors that constitute safe swallowing of food or liquid. Treatment of swallowing disorders, especially in adults, is not a matter of teaching swallowing in the sense of teaching a skill that a child has not yet acquired. The patient's previously well-managed swallowing skills are adversely affected because of the neurophysiological consequences of a disease process. The patient will have lost some of the skills involved in swallowing, but, of greater importance, the patient is simply unable to cope with the complex and pathological interactions taking place in the swallowing mechanism. The clinician's job, therefore, is to help the patient regain the skills to the extent possible, reduce the unfavorable interactions to the extent feasible, and to teach new and compensatory skills to the extent needed.

In terms of the knowledge base and skills manipulated, treatment of swallowing disorders differs from treatment of communication disorders. Nonetheless, a dynamic interaction between the clinician and the patient is common to both. As in the treatment of communication disorders, the clinician-patient interactions can be envisioned as planned relationships in which the clinician and the patient affect each other. Whether treatment of communication disorders or swallowing disorders, a single observation of a treatment session will convince us that in any treatment session, the clinician and the patient play out their respective roles and come out of successful treatment as changed persons. It is this view of treatment that has inspired these protocols.

If treatment is a set of scenarios in which the clinician and the patient play out their roles, protocols are scripts they follow to achieve improved patterns of safe swallowing. Therefore, the treatment sections in these protocols are written as scripts that help the clinician and the patient play their roles effectively, efficiently, and with a reasonable expectation of positive outcome for the patient and his or her family.

Another in a series of Plural Protocols, this book offers treatment protocols for dysphagia in adults. Although the book follows the general pattern established for treatment protocols, the current volume is designed both as a resource book on swallowing disorders and as protocols for treating those disorders.

These protocols for treating swallowing disorders in adults offer the background information and treatment overviews the clinician can use as resources. Advantages and disadvantages of various procedures are noted in the resource format. The actual treatments or exercises are written in the protocol format. It is expected that this combination of resource and protocol formats will help the clinician treat swallowing disorders effectively and efficiently.

By necessity, protocols are specific and appear prescriptive. However, all protocols, no matter how concrete they are in their precedural details, must be used with prudent clinical judgment. We expect these protocols to be used in a flexible manner that takes into consideration each individual patient's unique swallowing dynamics. Ultimately, it is the results of a careful assessment of the swallowing problems, the individual patient's strengths and limitations that will determine the nature of the treatment plan and its mode of implementation.

A companion volume entitled *Assessment of Dysphagia in Adults: Resources and Protocols in English and Spanish* also is available. This book, too, combines assessment resources and assessment protocols for the clinician to efficiently assess patients with dysphagia.

Acknowledgment

We would like to thank our families for their support and patience during this endeavor. We owe a special debt of gratitude to Fernando Arambula, whose technical help has been invaluable in completing this and the companion volume on dysphagia treatment. He has worked with the authors side by side and from day one to the deadline. Without his computer expertise and generous help with word processing and formatting, the two books would not have been completed on time. Thank you, thank you, Fernando, not only for your outstanding help but also for your gracious and cheerful support!

We would also like to thank Ines Isela Salinas who served as our Spanish language consultant for this project. She is a native of Mazatlán, Mexico where she received her professional education in nursing and worked as a registered nurse in a hospital setting. She also taught preventative medicine in Mazatlán, Mexico and Sinaloa, Mexico. For the past 6 years, she has been working as a Certified Nursing Assistant in the United States. She is currently working towards obtaining her license for registered nursing in the United States. Her expertise in Spanish as well as medical terminology has been invaluable in editing the Spanish sections of this book.

Introduction to Dysphagia Treatment Resources and Protocols

Treatment protocols are common in medicine, where such protocols are more prescriptive. Treatment plans in speech-language pathology and swallowing disorders need to be flexible and adaptable to individual patients. Nonetheless, clinical practice has identified a general pattern of treatment procedures that apply to many patients with swallowing disorders. Therefore, it is now possible to write specific protocols to address the various kinds of problems found in the different but dynamically related stages of safe swallow.

Treatment of swallowing disorders follows a thorough assessment of the patient's swallowing problems, strengths, and limitations. To make a competent assessment of patients with dysphagia and then to offer effective treatment, the clinician needs a insightful understanding of the neurophysiology of normal swallow, various diseases and disorders that negatively affect this vital function, specific disorders of swallowing, and the various means by which these disorders may be treated or clinically managed. A competently completed assessment will allow the speech-language pathologist to make recommendations for management and treatment of swallowing disorders. A complete set of bilingual assessment resources and protocols are offered in the companion volume entitled *Assessment of Dysphagia in Adults: Resources and Protocols in English and Spanish.*

Speech-language pathologists who assess and treat swallowing disorders in medical settings acquire a high level of proficiency through both academic coursework and practicum experiences under the guidance of knowledgeable and experienced clinicians. Although most students in graduate speech-language programs acquire the basic academic knowledge of swallowing and its disorders, their practicum experience in the assessment and treatment of dysphagia may be limited to one semester of medical externships. Students in some academic programs may not gain significant practicum experience in dysphagia. Those who wish to work in medical settings often depend on their clinical fellowship year (CFY) to gain valuable and in-depth practical experience in assessing and treating patients with dysphagia. It often is under the guidance of an expert supervisor that most graduate clinicians or master's degree holders gain the needed knowledge and skills in making a confident assessment of dysphagia and in implementing an effective treatment and management programs.

As with assessment of dysphagia, treatment often faces significant time pressures. There is always a certain amount of urgency about it, and the selected treatment strategies need to work right from the beginning. Depending on the assessment results and often on their own clinical experience and judgment as well, clinicians have to swiftly implement management and treatment strategies. Although implementation of these strategies is a team effort, speech-language pathologists tend to assume a critical leadership role in managing the typically multifaceted treatment program. Most experienced and expert clinicians accomplish this complex task deftly, often with no protocols in front of them. However, many beginning clinicians need detailed guidance and specific protocols that they can follow. They need step-by-step instructions, which may seem redundant to many experts and experienced clinicians. The rather large group of beginning practitioners includes not only graduate students but also CFY practitioners, newly certified and licensed clinicians, and other practitioners with many years of experience in assessing and treating communication disorders who are newly venturing into the unfamiliar territory of swallowing disorders, where they face risks unknown in their previous realm of professional practice. All of these clinicians need stepwise directions that spell out details. In training new clinicians, nothing can be taken for granted, because a simple mistake can lead to serious complications for the patient. In supervising beginning clinicians, we have found that in addition to details and specificity, repetition and self-contained protocols (sets of instructions or scenarios) are extremely important to train them to serve their patients well and to acquire not just acceptable professional skills but also exemplary expertise. Such clinicians cannot be expected to go back and forth in a resource manual or an assessment protocol to find information on steps to be taken and procedures to be implemented. Until they gain significant experience and expertise, clinicians need detailed protocols. All clinicians, however, can use the resources and abbreviated protocols that also are offered in this book. Clinicians at all stages and levels of practice, including the expert clinician, may find the detailed resources and protocols to be a much-needed reference source. It is with this perspective that we have written this book and its companion volume on treating and assessing dysphagia in adults.

Another perspective that has influenced the creation of this book, as well as the companion assessment book, is the increasing number of Spanish-speaking patients with swallowing disorders who are served by speech-language pathologists in the United States. Lack of systematic protocols and resources for bilingual clinicians has been a significant handicap in providing effective services to Spanish-speaking patients and their families. We have written this book and the assessment book to fill this great need for bilingual resources and protocols as well.

It is our clinical experience that instead of separate Spanish-language resources and protocols, a book that offers resources and protocols in English and Spanish arranged side by side will serve the practitioner better. We expect that most clinicians in the United States who work with Spanish-speaking patients are competent in English. Therefore, technical and background information directed to clinicians need not be in Spanish; however, information directed to the patients and their families need to be in both English and Spanish so that clinicians can offer relevant information in the language that is appropriate for the people they serve. Therefore, any resource material offered to patients and their families, instructions given to patients and their families, and assessment protocols are offered in both English and Spanish. Most protocols and resources are written in the split table format so that the bilingual clinician can always see both the Spanish and the English versions simultaneously. A monolingual English-speaking clinician serving only the English-speaking patient will not find anything complicated or cluttered; he or she simply can follow the English versions that are systematically laid out. We expect the bilingual clinicians to benefit from the dual-language presentation because they can cross-check the information offered in the two languages as they deliver instructions and implement treatment procedures. Above all, both bilingual and monolingual clinicians serving clients from either linguistic background will find easy-to-use treatment resources and protocols given in sufficient detail.

Organization of Dysphagia Treatment Resources and Protocols

The book is divided into seven sections. We offer two kinds of treatment information within this broad structure: background information, which includes a brief overview of treatment procedures, and protocols of treatment written in both English and Spanish. All treatment explanations or descriptions offered to the patient are in both languages. Similarly, all instructions given to the patient to implement various treatment exercises and strategies also are in both languages.

Section 1 of the book gives an overview of management and treatment of dysphagia. This section emphasizes the multidimensional nature of dysphagia intervention, offers suggestions for preparation for treatment, and gives an overview of treatment varieties. Section 2 offers a brief overview of general treatment or compensatory strategies that apply across swallowing disorders that affect different phases of swallow. Following this overview, the clinician will find general treatment and management strategies written in both English and Spanish.

The treatment strategies are grouped under the different stages of swallow. We recognize that discretely described physiological phases of swallow are dynamically connected in their functions, and that such discrete stages are more a matter of pedagogy than physiological reality. Nonetheless, from a practical standpoint, it is helpful to concentrate on the major locus of disorders for treatment of swallowing problems. Such major loci of disorders often may be found in somewhat arbitrarily described phases of normal swallow.

Section 3 includes treatment protocols for the oral preparatory phase disorders. After an overview of the phases and its disorders, the unit offers bilingual treatment protocols designed to increase oral sensitivity in patients with dysphagia, to improve the strength and tone of oral structures, and to increase the range of movement of the tongue, lips, and cheeks.

Bilingual protocols to treat the swallowing problems found in the oral phase of swallow are given in Section 4. The section begins with an overview of the phase and its disorders and moves on to protocols designed to increase oral sensitivity, improve the bolus movement, and minimize the risk of premature loss of the bolus.

Problems found in the pharyngeal phase of swallow and strategies to deal with them are the subject of Section 5. Bilingual treatment protocols are included to improve initiation of the pharyngeal swallow, reduce any residue in the valleculae and pharynx, and improve laryngeal closure and elevation.

Section 5 also briefly addresses swallowing problems associated with the esophageal phase of swallow. Speech-language pathologists do not directly treat problems associated with the esophageal phase of swallow. Nonetheless, they should be knowledgeable in these disorders and should make referrals to family physicians or gastroenterologists. Speech-language pathologists also can offer general strategies to the patient to manage the symptoms. A bilingual protocol with recommendations that may assist patients in managing problems associated with the esophageal phase is provided in this section.

Staff education in managing patients with swallowing problems is a significant part of speech-language pathologist's duties in medical and rehabilitation settings. Clinicians often spend a significant amount of their time assembling staff education information and protocols. To facilitate this important professional function, we have provided extensive resources to clinicians on staff education in Section 6. These bilingual resources include information that could be offered to various professional staff on safe feeding techniques, precautions to be taken, working with patients who have had head trauma, strokes, and so forth.

Section 7, the final in the book, is a compilation of valuable resources for patients, the nursing staff, and for posting safety related information in the patient's immediate environment. All important precautions the professional staff needs to take are included in the resources. Cautionary information in both Spanish and English are formatted in big and bold letters that are ready for printing and posting.

We trust that this bilingual book of resource and protocols will help the clinician to treat swallowing disorders using a systematic and detailed approach. Because of the combination of resources and protocols, the clinician will find, in this single source, information on and procedures for all aspects of dysphagia treatment.

How to Use the Accompanying CD

The CD that accompanies the book contains a variety of recording forms and treatment resources. All of the files on the CD are modifiable. The clinician can key in new information or delete nonapplicable material from the files. This will make it possible for the clinician to individualize the identifying information for particular clients he or she serves. The clinician can type in the name of the clinic, the clinician, the patient, the patient's family and address, and the treatment procedure offered. The forms thus modified and printed for the client's files will appear like the clinic stationery. While individualizing the recording sheets in this manner, the clinician can retain the standard recording sheet on the CD.

The personalized and printed forms will not look like the typical forms given in resource books. The modifiable and printable forms on the CD do not have page numbers, book chapter titles, and such other information that would make the forms inappropriate to place in a client's folder. Forms so modified and printed from the CD provided in the book will look like the practitioner's clinic stationery.

For the clinician's convenience, the CDs are prepared in simple Microsoft Word format that most people are familiar with; the CD is not encrypted in any way, to facilitate quick access and easy use of the documents it contains. Once again, the use of the CD will help the clinician save planning time and effort involved in getting prepared for treatment sessions.

Section 1

Overview of Management and Treatment of Dysphagia

Swallowing problems vary among patients according to the cause of the dysphagia and the nature and severity of the deficit. Therefore, each patient's individual needs must be assessed.

A comprehensive assessment accomplishes several objectives: First, assessment should lead to a description of the swallowing problems (diagnosis). Second, the assessment results should suggest a prognosis for the patient. Third, assessment outcomes should suggest a treatment plan for the patient. Fourth, the assessment results should help justify to the third party payers the requested reimbursement for services. This is why the speech-language pathologist must establish measurable and functional outcomes for dysphagia therapy. This chapter offers assistance to the speech-language pathologist in determining (a) prognosis for therapy, (b) components of a dysphagia treatment program, (c) preparation for therapy, and (d) types of therapy.

Establishing a Prognosis for Treatment

The clinician needs to consider several factors before initiating treatment for a patient. A prognostic statement can be determined by addressing the following questions:

- What is the patient's current diet?
- What type of dysphagia treatment should be offered?
- What is the patient's prognosis for improved swallowing (e.g., poor, guarded, fair, or good)?
- What is the patient's current cognitive status (e.g., is the patient able to follow directions)?
- Is the patient's family supportive?
- Is the patient motivated to participate in swallowing therapy?

Components of a Dysphagia Treatment Program

Dysphagia treatment is multidimensional and requires careful consideration of several factors such as the following (Logemann, 1998; Murry & Carrau, 2006; Perlman & Schulze-Delrieu, 1997; Swigert, 2000):

- The patient's strengths and weaknesses. A carefully designed treatment and management plan will describe what the patient is capable of, what he or she is not capable of, and what targets may realistically be achieved in treatment sessions.
- Treatment techniques that improve the patient's swallowing function, depending on the specific needs of the patient. An appropriate treatment plan will suggest specific treatment techniques that are selected to remediate a patient's particular swallowing problems.
- Education programs for family and staff. A comprehensive treatment, approach, or plan will include information and education for the family and professional staff in charge of the patient's care.
- Safe oral diet without putting the patient at risk for aspiration. The treatment plan should specify a range of diets that are safe for the patient.
- Plan of treatment that will improve the patient's quality of life. The treatment plan should be structured such that the overall goal of improving the quality of life for the patient is its essence.

Preparation for Treatment

In preparation for dysphagia treatment, it is important for the speech-language pathologist to consider the following (Swigert, 2000):

- Position of the patient. The patient should be sitting upright at as close as possible to a 90-degree angle for consuming foods or liquids, to decrease the risk of choking and aspiration.

- Precautions for positioning the patient. The clinician should be aware of any hip and limb precautions or head, neck, or spine surgery that the patient has undergone. The clinician could inadvertently cause injury to the patient if there is a specific positioning protocol in place for that patient. The clinician should check the patient's chart or ask the patient's nurse to obtain this information.

- Patient's current diet. To plan for dysphagia treatment, the clinician must know what food and liquid consistencies are safe for the patient to consume. This enables the clinician to introduce foods and liquids that are more advanced for the patient to manage. The patient's current diet can be obtained from the admitting physician's orders.

- Dietary precautions (e.g., diabetic, no-added-salt, fluid restriction). The clinician should know if the patient has dietary restrictions in order to plan for appropriate food or liquid presentations during treatment sessions. This information is available to the clinician on the admitting physician's orders or from the dietitian.

- Respiratory status (e.g., congestion, lung field sounds). The clinician should know the patient's respiratory status before initiation of dysphagia treatment. A baseline evaluation of the patient's lung fields is important if food or liquid presentations will be manipulated during the treatment. Respiratory status information can be found in the patient's progress notes or nurse's notes or obtained from the nurse.

- Cognitive status (e.g., alert and able to follow directions). The clinician should review the patient's progress notes to check the patient's level of alertness and the patient's response to directions as documented by nurses, physicians, and other therapists who have worked with the patient. The clinician should check the patient's cognitive status when initially assessing the patient.

- Patient participation in other therapies (e.g., occupational or physical therapy). The clinician should check to see if the patient has been cooperative with nursing staff or other therapists. This information can be obtained in the nursing or therapy daily progress notes.

- Temperature (e.g., high fever, low-grade fever). An elevated temperature or low-grade fever sometimes is a precursor to pneumonia. The clinician should check the patient's progress report to see if there is any documentation of an elevated temperature. The clinician can also ask the nurse.

- Weight (e.g., loss of weight). The clinician should check the patient's chart in the section on vital statistics or the weight record to see if there has been a significant weight loss of 5 pounds or more.

- Tolerance and endurance levels (e.g., can the patient tolerate 30 minutes of therapy?). The clinician should refer to the progress notes to see if comments have been made about the patient's tolerance and endurance and collaborate with other therapists who are working with the same patient. The clinician also should take note of the patient's tolerance and endurance level during the initial evaluation to determine if that patient is an appropriate candidate for speech therapy services.

Varieties of Treatment

Dysphagia treatment has various classifications. According to Logemann (1998), dysphagia therapy can be classified into two categories: (a) indirect therapy and (b) direct therapy.

Indirect therapy is used when the patient cannot safely consume an oral food or liquid diet. This kind of treatment does not include food. When incorporating indirect therapy into a treatment program, the speech-language pathologist may implement activities that address the following:

- Muscle control of the lips and tongue
- Muscle strength of the lips and the tongue
- Saliva swallows instead of actual attempts to swallow food
- Thermal-tactile stimulation activities

Direct therapy involves the presentation of oral trials of liquids and solids. The patient has to be safe on food or liquids to participate in direct therapy. In implementing direct therapy, the speech-language pathologist should include the following:

- Consistencies of food and liquids that are safe
- Specific directions to the patient while food or liquids are introduced
- Compensatory strategies for the patient to use during swallowing
- Instructions regarding specific amounts of food and liquids that are presented (e.g., ½ teaspoon versus 1 teaspoon at a time)

Dysphagia treatment techniques also may be classified as (a) compensatory strategies, (b) facilitation exercises, and (c) dietary changes (Swigert, 2000).

Compensatory strategies are used to compensate for the patient's swallowing disorder and involve actual eating. According to Swigert (2000), these strategies include the following:

- Posture changes (e.g., chin tuck, head turning)
- Sensory awareness strategies (e.g., thermal-tactile stimulation, sour bolus)
- Placement of food into the oral cavity (e.g., to the unaffected side of the patient's oral cavity)

Presentation of food (e.g., size and rate of food and liquids)

Facilitation exercises are used to improve muscle function (Swigert, 2000). These exercises are not used during meal times and include the following:

- Laryngeal adduction (e.g., pushing and pulling)
- Breath hold (Valsalva maneuver)

- Tongue hold
- Tongue base retraction
- Oral motor exercises
- Falsetto/pitch

Diet change techniques are used to alter the patient's diet for ease and safety in swallowing. According to Swigert (2000), these techniques address the following:

- Food texture (e.g., pureed, mechanical soft, or regular)
- Liquid consistency (e.g., regular versus thickened)
- Temperature of food (e.g., hot, cold, or room temperature)

Dysphagia therapy also can be classified as *compensatory swallow therapy* and *rehabilitative swallow therapy* (Murry & Carrau, 2006).

Compensatory swallow therapy techniques are used to strengthen control of the voluntary oral preparatory and oral phases of the swallow and include methods to stimulate the pharyngeal swallow. Compensatory swallow therapy techniques include exercises that do not require the patient to swallow foods and liquids. These techniques also are referred to as *indirect swallowing exercises*. These include the following:

- Oral-motor exercises
- Shaker exercise
- Thermal stimulation

Rehabilitative swallow therapy techniques are used to practice swallowing techniques and maneuvers and are used in combination with a variety of food consistencies and liquids. These techniques also are known collectively as *direct swallowing therapy* (Murry & Carrau, 2006). These include the following:

- Swallow maneuvers
  - Supraglottic swallow
  - Super-supraglottic swallow
  - Effortful swallow
  - Mendelsohn maneuver
  - Tongue hold maneuver

- Swallow postures
  - Head back
  - Chin down
  - Head rotated to damaged side
  - Chin down, head rotated to damaged side
  - Lying down on one side
  - Head tilt to damaged side
  - Head rotated

Treatment goals should address the reasons for the patient's swallowing difficulty. The speech-language pathologist should determine why the patient is having difficulty with the oral-pharyngeal phases of swallowing (e.g., why is there residue in the valleculae? why is there premature spillage before the swallow reflex has occurred? why is the patient pocketing food in the right side of the oral cavity?). The speech-language pathologist should request that a Modified Barium Videofluoroscopic Swallow Study (MBVSS), Fiberoptic Endoscopic Evaluation of Swallowing (FEES), or Flexible Endoscopic Evaluation of Swallowing with Sensory Testing (FEEST) be performed if a pharyngeal phase dysphagia is suspected. The information obtained solely from the clinical swallow examination cannot rule out aspiration. Therefore, speech-language pathologist who treat patients with suspected pharyngeal disorder in the absence of instrumental assessment place themselves and the patient at risk. However, there are situations in which only a clinical swallow examination can be completed because there is no access to an instrumental exam of the swallow (Swigert, 2000).

The speech-language pathologist needs to take all of the information that has been gathered in the assessment, select treatment targets that will improve the swallow, specify goals for each treatment phase, and implement treatment strategies that help accomplish the goals of treatment established for each patient.

The remainder of this book presents various treatment protocols that address the physiological problems that patients with dysphagia may exhibit. The treatment techniques are categorized into the following five areas:

1. General compensatory strategies
2. Oral preparatory techniques
3. Oral phase techniques
4. Pharyngeal phase techniques
5. Esophageal phase safe swallow instructions

Each treatment technique addresses (a) the problem, (b) general procedures for the clinician, (c) explanation to the patient in English and Spanish, (d) instructions to the patient in English and Spanish, and (e) potential advantages of the treatment technique.

It should be noted that these techniques constitute general guidelines for the speech-language pathologist. The clinician should always use clinical judgment and choose treatment techniques based on the particular patient profile established through a careful assessment of the patient's problems, strengths, and weaknesses.

Section 2

Management and Treatment of Dysphagia

General Treatment Procedures

Almost all patients with dysphagia need to compensate for their swallowing difficulties. Even if treatment is expected to be exceptionally effective, patients with dysphagia need to learn certain skills that help them compensate for their swallowing problems in the initial stages of treatment.

General treatment procedures may be used for patients with various types of dysphagia. These procedures have been grouped together in the protocols presented in this section. Protocols are provided for the following general treatment procedures:

- Cheek Push Strategy
- Mouth Rinse Strategy
- Strong Hold Food Strategy
- Multiple Swallow Strategy
- Alternating Solids and Liquids Strategy
- Empty Mouth Strategy

General Treatment Procedures
Protocol 2.1 (English/Spanish)
Cheek Push Strategy

As a general compensatory mechanism, the *Cheek Push Strategy* is used by the patient during mealtimes (Singh, Brockbank, Frost, & Tyler, 1995).

General Procedure
- The patient applies pressure to the outer cheek (this will remind the patient to check the inside of the cheek for pocketing of food).
- The patient repeats this strategy during meals.

Note to the Clinician
- Implement this strategy initially without presenting food to the patient.
- Introduce food as the patient progresses in therapy.

Potential Benefits of This Strategy
- Increased sensory awareness in the oral cavity
- Decreased pocketing of food or liquid

Protocol for Cheek Push Strategy: *Explanation and Instruction to the Patient*		
	Explanation in English	**Explicación en Español**
Clinician	This Cheek Push Strategy helps you decrease the amount of food or liquid that gets stuck in your cheeks.	Esta estrategia del empujón de la mejilla le ayuda a disminuir la cantidad de comida que se atora en sus mejillas.
	Instruction in English	**Instrucción in Español**
Clinician	1. Please apply pressure to the outer part of your right/left cheek [whichever side is affected]. 2. Please apply pressure on your cheek after each swallow that you take. 3. Please use this strategy after every swallow you take.	1. Por favor aplique presión a la parte de afuera de su mejilla derecha/izquierda [según el lado afectado]. 2. Por favor aplique presión en su mejilla después de cada trago que usted tome. 3. Por favor haga esta estrategia cada vez que usted trague.

General Treatment Procedures
Protocol 2.2 (English/Spanish)
Mouth Rinse Strategy

As a general compensatory mechanism, the *Mouth Rinse Strategy* is used by the patient after every meal.

General Procedures
- The patient rinses the mouth and spits after finishing a meal.
- The patient repeats this strategy after every meal.

Note to the Clinician
- Implement this strategy only with patients who are on the safest oral diet possible; the patient should be able to safely consume thin liquids (e.g., water).
- Use clinical judgment when deciding the appropriate time in treatment to implement this compensatory strategy.
- Make sure the patient understands the instructions.

Potential Benefits of This Strategy
- Increased sensory awareness of the oral cavity
- Decreased pocketing of food or liquids
- Decreased oral residue

Protocol for Mouth Rinse Strategy: *Explanation and Instruction to the Patient*		
	Explanation in English	**Explicación en Español**
Clinician	This Mouth Rinse Strategy helps you avoid food or liquid getting stuck inside your cheeks. This strategy may help increase the tension in your cheeks.	Esta estrategia del enjuago de la boca le ayudará asegurar que la comida o el líquido no se atore dentro de sus mejillas. Esta estrategia le ayudará a aumentar la tensión en sus mejillas.
	Instruction in English	**Instrucción en Español**
Clinician	1. Please take a sip of water out of the cup. 2. Please move the water around in your mouth without swallowing it. 3. Please move the water in your mouth for 1 minute. 4. Please spit the water out into the sink, after you have rinsed your mouth out. 5. Please do not swallow the water. 6. Please use this strategy at the end of every meal.	1. Por favor tome un sorbo de agua de la tasa. 2. Por favor mueva el agua alrededor en su boca sin tomársela. 3. Por favor mueva el agua en su boca por 1 minuto. 4. Por favor escupa el agua en el lava manos, después de que se enjuague su boca. 5. Por favor no se trague el agua. 6. Por favor use esta estrategia después de cada comida.

General Treatment Procedures
Protocol 2.3 (English/Spanish)

Strong Hold Food Strategy

As a general compensatory mechanism, the *Strong Hold Food Strategy* is used by the patient during mealtimes (Gangale, 1993; Logemann, 1998; Swigert, 2000).

General Procedures
- The patient should be on the safest oral diet for implementation of this compensatory strategy.
- The clinician or the patient places food on the stronger side of the tongue.
- The patient uses this strategy every time food is placed inside the mouth.

Potential Benefits of This Strategy
- Increased chewing skills
- Decreased pocketing of food

Protocol for Strong Hold Food Strategy: *Explanation and Instruction to the Patient*		
	Explanation in English	**Explicación en Español**
Clinician	This Strong Food Hold strategy helps avoid food or liquid getting stuck in the side of your cheek.	Esta estrategia de sostener fuerte la comida le ayudará a manejar la comida en su boca mientras que usted come.
	Instruction in English	**Instrucción en Español**
Clinician	1. Please put the food or liquid on the left/right side of your tongue [the stronger side of the tongue]. 2. Please chew your food on the same side as the one where I placed the food. 3. Please use this strategy every time you put food or liquid in your mouth.	1. Por favor ponga la comida o líquido en el lado derecho/izquierdo de su lengua [en el lado mas fuerte de la lengua]. 2. Por favor mastique su comida en el mismo lado donde puse la comida. 3. Por favor use esta estrategia cada vez que ponga comida o líquido en su boca.

General Treatment Procedures
Protocol 2.4 (English/Spanish)
Multiple Swallow Strategy

As a general compensatory mechanism, the *Multiple Swallow Strategy* is a set of procedures that are appropriate for the patient to use during mealtimes (Lazarus, Logemann, Rademaker, Kahrilas, Pajak, Lazar, & Halper, 1993; Silbergleit, Waring, Sullivan, & Maynard, 1991).

General Procedures
- The patient swallows multiple times (e.g., three times) after intake of one bolus of food.
- The patient repeats this strategy during mealtimes.

Potential Benefits of This Strategy
- Increased control of the bolus
- Decreased amount of food residue in the oral cavity

Protocol for Multiple Swallow Strategy: *Explanation and Instruction to the Patient*		
	Explanation in English	**Explicación en Español**
Clinician	This Multiple Swallow Strategy helps you clear everything in your mouth that was left after the first swallow.	Esta estrategia de tragos múltiples le ayudará a limpiar todo lo que se quedo en su boca después del primer trago.
	Instruction in English	**Instrucción en Español**
Clinician	1. Please take one bite of your food. 2. Please swallow two or three times before taking another bite. 3. Please use this strategy during all of your meals.	1. Por favor tome un bocado de comida. 2. Por favor trague dos o tres veces antes de que tome otro bocado. 3. Por favor use esta estrategia durante todas sus comidas.

General Treatment Procedures
Protocol 2.5 (English/Spanish)

Alternating Solids and Liquids Strategy

As a general compensatory mechanism, the *Alternating Solids and Liquids Strategy* is a set of procedures that is used by the patient during mealtimes (Logemann, 1998; Swigert, 2000).

General Procedures
- The patient takes a bite of food and then swallows.
- The patient takes a sip of liquid immediately after swallowing the food.
- The patient repeats this strategy during all meals.

Note to the Clinician
- Provide liquids and solids of varied consistencies.
- Use clinical judgment when presenting food with varied consistencies.

Potential Benefits of This Strategy
- Increased control of the bolus
- Decreased amount of food residue in the oral cavity

Protocol for Alternating Solids and Liquids: *Explanation and Instruction to the Patient*		
	Explanation in English	**Explicación en Español**
Clinician	This Alternating Solids and Liquids Food Strategy helps you clear everything in your mouth that was left after the first swallow.	Esta estrategia de alternar sólidos y líquidos le ayudará a limpiar todo lo que se quedo en la boca después del primer trago.
	Instruction in English	**Instrucción en Español**
Clinician	1. Please take one bite of food and swallow. 2. Now, please take a drink. 3. Now, please alternate between a bite of food and a drink of liquid. 4. Please continue to take a bite of food followed by a drink of liquid throughout your meal.	1. Por favor tome un bocado de comida y trague. 2. Luego, por favor tome un trago. 3. Luego, por favor alterne un bocado de comida y luego un trago de líquido. 4. Por favor continúe alternando un bocado de comida seguido con un trago de líquido hasta que se acabe su comida.

General Treatment Procedures
Protocol 2.6 (English/Spanish)

Empty Mouth Strategy

As a general compensatory mechanism, the *Empty Mouth Strategy* is a set of procedures used by the patient during mealtimes. The clinician should implement this strategy as needed in therapy (Boshart, 1998).

General Procedures

- The patient does not take another bite of food unless the mouth is completely empty.
- The clinician gives verbal cues to ensure that there is nothing inside the mouth before the patient places more food or liquid into it.
- The clinician repeats the verbal cues to the patient throughout the meal.
- The clinician instructs the patient, caregiver, or nursing staff to give such verbal cues.

Potential Benefits of This Strategy

- Decreased risk for aspiration due to a delayed swallow reflex
- Decreased presence of oral residue

Protocol for Empty Mouth Strategy: *Explanation and Instruction to the Patient*		
	Explanation in English	**Explicación en Español**
Clinician	This Empty Mouth Strategy helps you clear your mouth. This strategy may help you keep food or liquid from going inside your lungs.	Esta estrategia de la boca vacía le ayudará a limpiar su boca. Esta estrategia le ayudara a prevenir que la comida o líquidos no entren a los pulmones.
	Instruction in English	**Instrucción en Español**
Clinician	1. Please put some food in your mouth.	1. Por favor ponga la comida en su boca.
	2. Now, please swallow your food completely.	2. Luego, por favor trague su comida completamente.
	3. After you swallow, please make sure that there is not any food or liquid left inside your mouth.	3. Después de que trague, por favor este seguro que no ha dejado comida o líquido en su boca.
	4. Please put more food in your mouth only when your mouth is completely empty of food.	4. Por favor ponga mas comida en su boca solamente cuando su boca este completamente vacía de comida.
	5. Please use this strategy during all of your meals.	5. Por favor use esta estrategia durante todas sus comidas.

Section 3

Treatment for Oral Preparatory Phase Disorders

Overview of the Oral Preparatory Phase of Swallowing and Associated Disorders

In developing an appropriate management program for patients with dysphagia, the speech-language pathologist should consider the following: (a) components of the oral preparatory phase, (b) problems associated with the oral preparatory phase, (c) signs and symptoms of oral preparatory phase disorders, and (d) general treatment goals. These strategies include compensatory swallowing therapy exercises and rehabilitative swallow therapy strategies.

Components of the Oral Preparatory Phase

The oral preparatory phase consists of the following skills:

- Placement of food into the mouth
- Closure of the lips to create a lip seal
- Movement of the tongue laterally to push the food onto the teeth for the patient to chew
- Movement of the tongue vertically to break down the bolus
- Formation of the bolus to prepare for swallowing
- Control of the tongue needed to form and manage the bolus

Physiological and Neuromotor Deficiencies in the Oral Preparatory Phase

Patients with dysphagia may exhibit one or more of the following physiological and neuromotor problems during the oral preparatory phase of the swallow:

- Decreased sensitivity of the oral cavity to hot temperatures
- Decreased sensitivity of the oral cavity to cold temperatures
- Decreased muscle strength of the lips
- Decreased range of motion of the lips
- Decreased tongue strength
- Decreased range of motion of the tongue
- Reduced tongue elevation
- Reduced lateral tongue movement
- Decreased cheek strength

Swallowing Disorders Associated with the Oral Preparatory Phase

Patient may exhibit one or more of the following signs and symptoms of dysphagia due to the physiological and neuromotor problems associated with the oral preparatory phase of the swallow:

- Loss of food or liquid outside of the oral cavity
- Pocketing of food or liquid inside the cheeks
- Increased drooling

General Treatment Goals for Patients with Oral Preparatory Phase Disorders

Treatment for oral preparatory phase disorders addresses altered sensory awareness in the oral region, decreased strength and range of motion of the oral structures, reduced efficiency in bolus formation, and inadequate hold of the bolus and incorporates the following goals:

- Increasing sensory awareness of the lips, cheeks, and tongue
- Increasing lip, tongue, and cheek strength and range of motion
- Improving the bolus formation in the mouth
- Improving an adequate hold of the bolus

The protocols that follow address these concerns regarding the oral preparatory phase of the swallow.

Treatment for Oral Preparatory Phase Disorders
Increasing Oral Sensitivity

Overview

Many patients who present for treatment of dysphagia related to the oral preparatory phase of swallow exhibit decreased sensitivity in the oral cavity. This may be secondary to tactile agnosia for food, swallow apraxia, delayed onset of the oral swallow, or delayed trigger of the swallow (Logemann, 1998).

The following treatment protocols are provided to increase oral sensitivity in patients with dysphagia (Boshart, 1998; Gangale, 1993; Logemann, 1993; Logemann, Pauloski, Colangelo, Lazarus, Fujiu, & Kahrilas, 1995; Murry & Carrau, 2006; Swigert, 2000):

- Cold Lip Rub
- Warm Lip Rub
- Soft Lip Press
- Bitter Press
- Iced Cheek Technique
- Washcloth Rub
- Cold Inner Cheek Rub
- Toothbrush Rub
- Tongue Tickle
- Back Tongue Tickle

Treatment for Oral Preparatory Phase Disorders
Increasing Oral Sensitivity
Protocol 3.1 (English/Spanish)

Cold Lip Rub

The *Cold Lip Rub* is a set of procedures used to increase sensory awareness in the lips (Murry & Carrau, 2006).

General Procedures
- Moisten the patient's lips with a Toothette sponge before performing this exercise.
- "Wring out" the Toothette sponge before applying moisture to the patient's lips.
- Use a teaspoon that has been placed in the freezer for at least an hour.
- Place the back of the spoon on the patient's lips to stimulate them.
- Use mild to moderate pressure when applying the spoon to the patient's lips.

Potential Benefits of This Exercise
- Increased oral sensory awareness
- Increased stimulation of the labial muscles

Protocols for Cold Lip Rub: *Explanation and Instruction to the Patient*		
	Explanation in English	**Explicación en Español**
Clinician	The Cold Lip Rub exercise helps you to increase sensory awareness in your lips.	Este ejercicio de El Roce Frió al Labio le ayuda a aumentar el conocimiento sensorial de sus labios.
	Instruction in English	**Instrucción en Español**
Clinician	1. I will moisten your lips with a Toothette sponge. 2. Next, I will put a cold teaspoon on your lips. 3. Then I will apply pressure on your lips with the spoon.	1. Voy a mojarle los labios con una esponjita. 2. Luego, voy a ponerle una cucharilla fría en sus labios. 3. Voy aplicarle presión en sus labios con una cucharilla.

Treatment for Oral Preparatory Phase Disorders
Increasing Oral Sensitivity
Protocol 3.2 (English/Spanish)

Warm Lip Rub

The *Warm Lip Rub* is a set of procedures used to increase sensory awareness in the lips (Gangale, 1993).

General Procedures
- Moisten the patient's lips with a wet Toothette sponge; oftentimes, the patient's lips are dry.
- "Wring out" the Toothette sponge before applying moisture to the patient's lips; otherwise, the excess moisture may decrease the effect of the warm teaspoon.
- Place a teaspoon into warm water 5 minutes before the treatment session.
- Apply the warmed teaspoon to the patient's lips using mild to moderate pressure.
- Never use hot water to warm the teaspoon!

Potential Benefits of This Exercise
- Increased sensory awareness of the lips
- Increased stimulation of the labial muscles

Protocols for Warm Lip Rub: *Explanation and Instruction to the Patient*		
	Explanation in English	**Explicación en Español**
Clinician	The Warm Lip Rub Exercise helps you to increase sensation in your lips.	Este Ejercicio de el Roce Tibio al Labio le ayuda a aumentar la sensación en sus labios.
	Instruction in English	**Instrucción en Español**
Clinician	1. I will moisten your lips with a sponge. 2. Next, I will place a warm teaspoon on your lips with a little bit of pressure. 3. I will repeat this exercise 10 times.	1. Voy a mojarle los labios con una esponjita. 2. Luego, voy a ponerle una cucharilla tibia en sus labios usando poca presión. 3. Voy a repetir este ejercicio 10 veces.

Treatment for Oral Preparatory Phase Disorders
Increasing Oral Sensitivity
Protocol 3.3 (English/Spanish)

Soft Lip Press

The *Soft Lip Press* is a set of procedures used to increase sensory awareness in the lips (Boshart, 1998; Murry & Carrau, 2006).

General Procedures
- Using a Toothette sponge, gloved finger, or soft-bristle toothbrush, apply pressure to the patient's upper lip; then apply pressure to the patient's lower lip.
- Apply pressure in a circular pattern across the lips.

Potential Benefits of This Exercise
- Increased sensory awareness of the upper and lower lips
- Increased lip closure

Protocols for Soft Lip Press: *Explanation and Instruction to the Patient*		
	Explanation in English	**Explicación en Español**
Clinician	The Soft Lip Press Exercise helps you increase the sensation in your lips.	Este Ejercicio la Presión Suave al Labio le ayuda a aumentar la sensación en sus labios.
	Instruction in English	**Instrucción en Español**
Clinician	1. I will place a sponge/my finger/soft toothbrush/ on your upper lip.	1. Voy a ponerle una esponja/mi dedo/un cepillo de dientes suave en su labio de arriba.
	2. I will apply mild to deep pressure to your upper lip.	2. Voy aplicar presión poco severo a profundo en su labio de arriba.
	3. I will apply pressure across your upper lip 10 times.	3. Voy aplicarle presión sobre todo su labio de arriba 10 veces.
	4. I will place a sponge/my finger/soft toothbrush on your lower lip.	4. Voy a ponerle una esponja/mi dedo/un cepillo de dientes suave en su labio de abajo.
	5. I will apply mild to deep pressure to your lower lip.	5. Voy aplicarle presión poco severa a profunda en su labio de abajo.
	6. I will apply pressure across your lower lip 10 times.	6. Voy aplicarle presión sobre su labio de abajo 10 veces.

Treatment for Oral Preparatory Phase Disorders
Increasing Oral Sensitivity
Protocol 3.4 (English/Spanish)

Bitter Press

The *Bitter Press* is a set of procedures used to increase sensory awareness in the lips (Gangale, 1993; Logemann, Pauloski, Colangelo, Lazarus, Fujiu, & Kahrilas, 1995).

General Procedures
- Take a frozen lemon glycerin swab or a Q-tip that has been dipped in lemon juice and apply it to the patient's upper lip.
- Apply the Q-tip or lemon glycerin swab to the patient's lower lip.
- Use mild to deep pressure across the upper and lower lips in a circular movement.
- Complete 10 trials of this exercise across the upper and lower lips.

Potential Benefits of This Exercise
- Increased sensory awareness in the upper and lower lips
- Increased muscle stimulation of the upper and lower lips

Protocols for Bitter Press: *Explanation and Instruction to the Patient*		
	Explanation in English	**Explicación en Español**
Clinician	This Bitter Press exercise helps you increase the sensation in your lips. This exercise may help stimulate the muscles in your lips.	Este ejercicio la Presión Amarga le ayuda a aumentar la sensación en sus labios. Este ejercicio puede ayudarle a estimular los músculos en sus labios.
	Instruction in English	**Instrucción en Español**
Clinician	1. I will place a Q-tip/sponge on your upper lip. 2. The Q-tip or sponge may taste sour. 3. I will apply mild to deep pressure across your upper lip. 4. I will apply pressure across your upper lip 10 times. 5. I will place a Q-tip/sponge on your lower lip. 6. The Q-tip or sponge may taste sour. 7. I will apply mild to deep pressure across your lower lip. 8. I will apply pressure across your lower lip 10 times.	1. Voy a ponerle una esponja en su labio de arriba. 2. La esponja tal vez sepa agria. 3. Voy aplicarle presión poco severa a profunda sobre su labio de arriba. 4. Voy aplicarle presión sobre su labio de arriba 10 veces. 5. Voy a ponerle una esponja en su labio de abajo. 6. La esponja tal vez sepa agria. 7. Voy aplicarle presión poco severa a profunda sobre su labio de abajo. 8. Voy aplicarle presión sobre su labio de abajo 10 veces.

Treatment for Oral Preparatory Phase Disorders
Increasing Oral Sensitivity
Protocol 3.5 (English/Spanish)
Iced Cheek Technique

The *Iced Cheek Technique* is a set of procedures used to increase sensory awareness in the cheeks (Gangale, 1993).

General Procedures
- Use a glove filled with ice or a small ice pack.
- Place the iced glove or ice pack on the right corner of the patient's mouth.
- Slide the iced glove or ice pack backward from the right corner of the patient's mouth toward the cheekbone.
- Wipe the patient's cheek with a towel after each trial.
- Wait 30 seconds before beginning the next trial.
- Complete 10 trials of this strategy; then repeat the exercise on the left side of the patient's face.

Potential Benefits of This Exercise
- Increased sensory awareness of the right and left cheeks
- Increased muscle stimulation of the right and left cheeks

Protocols for Iced Cheek Technique: *Explanation and Instruction to the Patient*		
	Explanation in English	**Explicación en Español**
Clinician	This Iced Cheek Technique helps you increase sensation in your cheeks. This exercise may stimulate the muscles in your cheeks.	Este Técnico de Mejilla Helada le ayuda a aumentar sensación en sus mejillas. Este ejercicio también le estímula los músculos en sus mejillas.
	Instruction in English	**Instrucción en Español**
Clinician	1. I will place an ice pack/glove filled with ice on the right corner of your upper lip. 2. I will slide the ice pack/glove filled with ice backward toward the upper part of your cheek. 3. I will apply the ice pack/glove filled with ice on your cheek 10 times. 4. I will place the ice pack/glove filled with ice on the left corner of your upper lip. 5. I will slide the ice pack/glove filled with ice backward toward the upper part of your cheek. 6. I will apply the ice pack/glove filled with ice to your cheek 10 times.	1. Voy a ponerle una bolsa/guante lleno de hielo en la esquina derecha de su labio de arriba. 2. Voy a resbalar la bolsa/guante lleno de hielo hacia atrás para la parte de arriba de su mejilla. 3. Voy aplicar la bolsa/guante lleno de hielo 10 veces a su mejilla. 4. Voy a ponerle una bolsa/guante lleno de hielo en la esquina izquierda de su labio de arriba. 5. Voy a resbalar la bolsa/guante lleno de hielo hacia atrás para la parte de arriba de su mejilla. 6. Voy aplicar la bolsa/guante lleno de hielo 10 veces a su mejilla.

Treatment for Oral Preparatory Phase Disorders
Increasing Oral Sensitivity
Protocol 3.6 (English/Spanish)

Washcloth Rub

The *Washcloth Rub* is a set of procedures used to increase sensory awareness in the lips and cheeks (Gangale, 1993).

General Procedures
- Take a washcloth and rub the patient's face (especially the cheeks and lips).
- Avoid the patient's eyes or nose with the washcloth.
- Apply large pressing motions across the face.
- Alternate the use of warm and cold washcloths on the patient's face.
- Repeat this exercise 10 times, alternating warm and cold washcloths, or as tolerated by the patient.

Potential Benefits of This Exercise
- Increased sensory awareness in the lips
- Increased sensory awareness in the cheeks

Protocols for Washcloth Rub: *Explanation and Instruction to the Patient*		
	Explanation in English	**Explicación en Español**
Clinician	The Washcloth Rub exercise helps increase the sensation in your face and lips. This exercise may help stimulate the muscles in your lips and cheeks.	Este ejercicio de El Roce con Toallita le ayuda a aumentar la sensación de su cara y labios. Este ejercicio puede ayudarle a estimular los músculos de sus labios y mejillas.
	Instruction in English	**Instrucción en Español**
Clinician	1. I will place a cold washcloth on your face and rub your face with the wash cloth gently. 2. You will feel a cold washcloth and then a warm washcloth applied to your face. 3. You will feel moderate pressure on your face during this exercise. 4. I will not put the washcloth near your eyes or nose. 5. I will apply a cold wash to your face and then a warm washcloth. 6. I will repeat this exercise 10 times, alternating warm and cold washcloths.	1. Voy a ponerle una toalla mojada y fría en su cara y le voy a frotar su cara con la toalla suavemente. 2. Tal vez sienta una toalla fría y luego una toalla tibia que se aplica a su cara. 3. Va ha sentir presión moderada en su cara durante este ejercicio. 4. No le pondré la toalla cerca de sus ojos o nariz. 5. Le aplicare una toalla mojada y fría a su cara y luego una toalla tibia. 6. Voy a repetir este ejercicio 10 veces, alternando toallas tibias y frías.

Treatment for Oral Preparatory Phase Disorders
Increasing Oral Sensitivity
Protocol 3.7 (English/Spanish)

Cold Inner Cheek Rub

The *Cold Inner Cheek Rub* is a set of procedures used to increase sensory awareness in the cheeks (Logemann, 1998).

General Procedures
- Use an iced spoon or a frozen lemon glycerin swab.
- Insert a tongue depressor inside the patient's cheek and pull the cheek gently outward.
- Use the other hand to apply the frozen lemon glycerin swab or cold teaspoon to the patient's inner cheek.
- Apply gentle pressure, using circular or back-and-forth movements.
- Repeat five trials on each cheek, or as many trials as the patient tolerates.

Potential Benefits of This Exercise
- Increased sensory awareness in the right and left cheeks
- Increased muscle stimulation in the right and left cheeks
- Increased overall muscle tone in both the left and right cheeks

Protocols for Cold Inner Cheek Rub: *Explanation and Instruction to the Patient*		
	Explanation in English	**Explicación en Español**
Clinician	This Cold Inner Cheek Rub exercise helps to increase the sensation in the inner part of your cheek. This exercise may help stimulate the muscles in your inner cheek.	Este ejercicio de El Roce Frió del Interior de la Mejilla le ayuda a aumentar la sensación por dentro de la mejilla. Este ejercicio puede ayudarle a estimular los músculos de adentro de la mejilla.
	Instruction in English	**Instrucción en Español**
Clinician	1. I will put a tongue depressor in the right side of your mouth and pull your cheek gently outward. 2. I will put a cold teaspoon/Q-tip in your mouth. 3. I will rub the inside of your right cheek with the teaspoon/Q-tip. 4. I will rub the inside of your right cheek five times. 5. I will put a tongue depressor in the left side of your mouth and pull your cheek gently outward. 6. I will put a cold teaspoon/Q-tip in your mouth. 7. I will rub the inside of your left cheek with the teaspoon/Q-tip. 8. I will rub the inside of your left cheek five times.	1. Voy a poner un depresor de lengua en el lado derecho de su boca y voy a estirar su mejilla suavemente para afuera. 2. Voy a poner una cuchara fría en su boca. 3. Voy a tallar lo de adentro de su mejilla derecha con una cuchara. 4. Le tallaré lo de adentro de la mejilla derecha cinco veces. 5. Voy a poner un depresor de lengua en el lado izquierdo su boca y voy a estirar su mejilla suavemente hacia afuera. 6. Voy a poner una cuchara fría en su boca. 7. Voy a tallarle lo de adentro de su mejilla izquierda con una cuchara. 8. Le tallaré lo de adentro de su mejilla izquierda cinco veces.

Treatment for Oral Preparatory Phase Disorders
Increasing Oral Sensitivity
Protocol 3.8 (English/Spanish)

Toothbrush Rub

The *Toothbrush Rub* is a set of procedures used to increase sensory awareness in the tongue (Boshart, 1998; Gangale, 1993).

General Procedures
- Use a toothbrush, Toothette, or lemon glycerin swab.
- Place the toothbrush, Toothette, or lemon glycerin swab on the right side of the patient's posterior tongue.
- Slide the toothbrush, Toothette, or lemon glycerin swab from the posterior portion of the tongue to the tip of the tongue on the right side.
- Alternate this exercise from the right side of the tongue to the left side of the tongue.
- Repeat this exercise 10 times or as tolerated by the patient.

Potential Benefits of This Exercise
- Increased sensory awareness on the right and left side of the tongue
- Increased stimulation of the tongue muscles on the right and left sides

Protocols for Toothbrush Rub: *Explanation and Instruction to the Patient*		
	Explanation in English	**Explicación en Español**
Clinician	The Toothbrush Rub exercise helps to increase the sensory awareness of your tongue. This exercise may help stimulate the muscles in your tongue.	Este ejercicio de El Roce del Cepillo de Dientes aumenta el conocimiento sensatorio de su lengua. Este ejercicio puede ayudarle a estimular los músculos de su lengua.
	Instruction in English	**Instrucción en Español**
Clinician	1. I will put a toothbrush/Toothette swab/lemon glycerin swab on the back part of the right side of your tongue. 2. I will rub the right side of your tongue starting at the back of your tongue and move toward the front of your tongue. 3. I will rub the right side of your tongue five times. 4. I will put a toothbrush/Toothette swab/lemon glycerin swab on the back part of the left side of your tongue. 5. I will rub the left side of your tongue starting at the back of your tongue and move toward the front of your tongue. 6. I will rub the left side of your tongue five times. 7. I will rub the top of your tongue with a toothbrush/Toothette swab/lemon glycerin swab. 8. I will begin at the back center of your tongue and move forward toward the tip of your tongue. 9. I will rub the top of your tongue five times.	1. Voy a poner un cepillo de dientes/ una esponjita/un aplicador de limón y glicerina en la parte de atrás del lado derecho de su lengua. 2. Voy a tallar el lado derecho de su lengua comenzando con lo atrás de su lengua y moviéndome al frente de su lengua. 3. Le tallare el lado derecho de su lengua cinco veces. 4. Voy a poner un cepillo de dientes/ una esponjita/ un aplicador de limón y glicerina en la parte de atrás del lado izquierdo de su lengua. 5. Voy a tallarle el lado izquierdo de su lengua comenzando con la parte de atrás de su lengua y moviéndome hacia el frente de su lengua. 6. Le voy a tallar el lado izquierdo de su lengua cinco veces. 7. Le voy a tallar lo de arriba de su lengua con un cepillo de dientes/ una esponjita/un aplicador de limón y glicerina. 8. Voy a comenzar en la parte de atrás de su lengua y moverme hacia el frente a la punta de su lengua. 9. Le tallare lo de arriba de su lengua cinco veces.

Treatment for Oral Preparatory Phase Disorders
Increasing Oral Sensitivity
Protocol 3.9 (English/Spanish)

Tongue Tickle

The *Tongue Tickle* is a set of procedures used to increase sensory awareness (Boshart, 1998).

General Procedures
- Use a tongue depressor and apply it to the right side of the patient's tongue tip.
- Move the tongue depressor along the lateral margins of the tongue to the left side.
- Use gentle rubbing strokes laterally from right to left.
- Repeat this exercise 10 times.
- Repeat this exercise from the left to the right side of the tongue.

Potential Benefits of This Exercise
- Increased sensory awareness of the left and right sides of the tongue
- Increased stimulation of the right and left sides of the tongue muscles

Protocols for Tongue Tickle: *Explanation and Instruction to the Patient*		
	Explanation in English	**Explicación en Español**
Clinician	This Tongue Tickle exercise will help you increase the sensation and strength of your tongue.	Este ejercicio de El Cosquilleo de Lengua le ayudará a aumentar la sensación y fuerza de su lengua.
	Instruction in English	**Instrucción en Español**
Clinician	1. I will place a tongue depressor on the tip of your tongue. 2. I will rub the tip of your tongue with the tongue depressor, moving from the right to the left side. 3. You will feel a tickling sensation on your tongue. 4. I will repeat this exercise 10 times. 5. I will place the tongue depressor on the tip of your tongue. 6. I will rub the tip of your tongue with the tongue depressor, moving from the left to the right side. 7. You will feel a tickling sensation on your tongue. 8. I will repeat this exercise 10 times.	1. Voy a ponerle un depresor de lengua en la punta de su lengua. 2. Voy a tallarle la punta de su lengua con el depresor, moviéndolo de la derecha a la izquierda. 3. Tal vez sienta una sensación de cosquillo en su lengua. 4. Voy a repetir este ejercicio 10 veces. 5. Voy a ponerle un depresor de lengua en la punta de su lengua. 6. Voy a tallarle la punta de su lengua con un depresor, moviéndolo de la izquierda a la derecha. 7. Tal vez sienta una sensación de cosquillo en su lengua. 8. Voy a repetir este ejercicio 10 veces.

Treatment for Oral Preparatory Phase Disorders
Increasing Oral Sensitivity
Protocol 3.10 (English/Spanish)

Back Tongue Tickle

The *Back Tongue Tickle* is a set of procedures used to increase sensory awareness of the tongue (Boshart, 1998).

General Procedures
- Use a Q-tip (that has been placed in ice), tongue depressor, or Toothette sponge.
- Place one of these devices at the tip of the patient's tongue and move it posteriorly toward the dorsum of the tongue.
- Repeat this exercise five times or as tolerated by the patient.

Potential Benefits of This Exercise
- Increased sensory awareness in the tongue
- Increased stimulation of the tongue muscles

Protocols for Back Tongue Tickle: *Explanation and Instruction to the Patient*		
	Explanation in English	**Explicación en Español**
Clinician	This Back Tongue Tickle exercise helps you increase sensation on the back part of your tongue. This exercise may help stimulate the muscles in the back of your tongue.	Este ejercicio de EL Cosquilleo de la Lengua Posterior le ayuda a aumentar la sensación de la parte de atrás de su lengua. Este ejercicio puede ayudarle a estimular los músculos de atrás de su lengua.
	Instruction in English	**Instrucción en Español**
Clinician	1. I want you to open your mouth wide. 2. I will apply pressure with a tongue depressor at the tip of your tongue. 3. I will move the tongue depressor from the tip of your tongue to the back of your tongue. 4. I will repeat this exercise 10 times.	1. Quiero que abra su boca ancha. 2. Voy aplicarle presión con un depresor de lengua a la punta de su lengua. 3. Voy a mover el depresor de la punta de su lengua hacia atrás de su lengua. 4. Voy a hacer este ejercicio 10 veces.

Treatment for Oral Preparatory Phase Disorders Improving the Strength and Range of Movement of the Lips and Cheeks

Overview

Many patients who need treatment for dysphagia have difficulty keeping food and liquid in the oral cavity. The food and liquid placed in the mouth tend to fall out. This problem may be secondary to decreased strength and range of movement in the lips and cheeks. Therefore, the speech-language pathologist should offer exercises that help improve the strength and range of movement of the lips and cheeks.

Protocols are provided for compensatory swallow therapy techniques that can help increase the strength and range of movement of the lips and cheeks. These exercises are expected to decrease spillage of food or liquids outside of the oral cavity (Boshart, 1998; Gangale, 1993; Logemann, 1998; Murry & Carrau, 2006).

- Lip Squeeze Exercise
- Lip Rub Exercise
- Lower Lip Push-up Exercise
- Close/Open Lip Exercise
- Pucker and Smile Exercise
- Tight Lip Exercise
- Big Smile Exercise
- Cheek Puff Exercise

Treatment for Oral Preparatory Phase Disorders
Strengthening the Lips
Protocol 3.11 (English/Spanish)

Lip Squeeze Exercise

The *Lip Squeeze Exercise* is a set of procedures used to increase lip closure, to decrease spillage of food or liquid outside of the oral cavity (Boshart, 1998; Murry & Carrau, 2006).

General Procedures
- Instruct the patient to squeeze and tighten the lips together.
- Have the patient hold the lips together for 3 seconds; then have the patient relax.
- Repeat 10 trials of this exercise or as many trials that the patient can tolerate.

Potential Benefits of This Exercise
- Increased muscle strength of the lips
- Increased sensory awareness of the lips
- Decreased drooling

Protocols for Lip Squeeze Exercise: *Explanation and Instruction to the Patient*		
	Explanation in English	**Explicación en Español**
Clinician	This Lip Squeeze Exercise helps you increase the strength in your lips to prevent food or liquid from falling out of your mouth, while you are eating or drinking.	Este Ejercicio de Apretar los Labios le ayuda a aumentar la fuerza de sus labios para evitar que la comida o líquido se salga de la boca, mientras que come o toma.
	Instruction in English	**Instrucción en Español**
Clinician	1. Please squeeze and tighten your lips together. 2. Please hold your lips in this position for 3 seconds. 3. Please let go and relax. 4. Please do this exercise 10 times.	1. Por favor apriete sus labios juntos. 2. Por favor retenga esta posición con sus labios por 3 segundos. 3. Por favor afloje los labios y descanse. 4. Por favor haga este ejercicio 10 veces.

Treatment for Oral Preparatory Phase Disorders
Strengthening the Lips
Protocol 3.12 (English/Spanish)

Lip Rub Exercise

The *Lip Rub Exercise* is a set of procedures used to increase lip closure, to decrease spillage of liquid or food outside of the oral cavity (Boshart, 1998).

General Procedures
- Put lip moisturizer/petroleum jelly on the patient's lips
- Instruct the patient to rub the lips together.
- Repeat this exercise 10 times or as tolerated.

Potential Benefits of This Exercise
- Increased lip strength
- Increased sensory awareness of the lips
- Increased lip tone
- Increased range of motion of the lips
- Decreased drooling

Protocols for Lip Rub Exercise: *Explanation and Instruction to the Patient*		
	Explanation in English	**Explicación en Español**
Clinician	This Lip Rub Exercise helps to increase the strength and tone in the muscles of your lips. This exercise may help you to keep food or liquid from spilling outside of your mouth.	Este Ejercicio de El Roce de Labios le ayuda a aumentar la fuerza y tono en los músculos de sus labios. Este ejercicio puede ayudarle a guardar que la comida o líquido no se derrame fuera de su boca.
	Instruction in English	**Instrucción en Español**
Clinician	1. I will put some lip moisturizer/ petroleum jelly on your lips. 2. Please rub your lips together. 3. I will do this exercise 10 times.	1. Voy a ponerle crema hidratante para los labios/pomada en sus labios. 2. Por favor flote sus labios juntos. 3. Por favor haga este ejercicio 10 veces.

Treatment for Oral Preparatory Phase Disorders
Strengthening the Lips
Protocol 3.13 (English/Spanish)

Lower Lip Push-up Exercise

The *Lower Lip Push-up Exercise* is a set of procedures used to increase lip closure, to decrease spillage of food or liquid outside of the oral cavity (Gangale, 1993).

General Procedures
- Instruct the patient to move the lower lip upward until it completely covers the upper lip.
- Complete 10 trials of this exercise.

Potential Benefits of This Exercise
- Increased lip strength
- Increased lip tone
- Increased sensory awareness in the lips
- Increased range of motion of the lips
- Increased lip closure
- Decreased drooling

Protocols for Lower Lip Push-up Exercise: *Explanation and Instruction to the Patient*		
	Explanation in English	**Explicación en Español**
Clinician	This Lower Lip Push-up Exercise helps to increase the strength and tone in your lips. This exercise may help you to close your lips without food or liquid falling out.	Este Ejercicio de Levantar el Labio Inferior le ayuda a aumentar la fuerza y tono de sus labios. Este ejercicio puede ayudarle a cerrar sus labios sin que la comida o líquido se tire.
	Instruction in English	**Instrucción en Español**
Clinician	1. Please move your lower lip upward and cover your upper lip with your lower lip. 2. Please repeat this exercise 10 times.	1. Por favor mueva su labio de abajo hacia arriba y cubra su labio de arriba con el labio de abajo. 2. Por favor haga este ejercicio 10 veces.

Treatment for Oral Preparatory Phase Disorders
Strengthening the Lips
Protocol 3.14 (English/Spanish)

Close/Open Lip Exercise

The *Close/Open Lip Exercise* is a set of procedures used to increase lip closure, to decrease spillage of food or liquid outside of the oral cavity (Murry & Carrau, 2006).

General Procedures
- Make sure that the patient has adequate nasal airway patency before implementing any treatment technique.
- Instruct the patient to open the mouth wide and then close it.
- Tell the patient to press the lips together firmly and hold that position for 3 seconds.
- Repeat 10 trials of this exercise.

Potential Benefits of This Exercise
- Increased lip strength
- Increased awareness of lips
- Increased lip closure
- Decreased drooling

Protocols for Close/Open Lip Exercise: *Explanation and Instruction to the Patient*		
	Explanation in English	**Explicación en Español**
Clinician	This Close/Open Lip Exercise helps increase the strength, tone, and movement of your lips. This exercise may help prevent food or liquid from spilling out of your mouth.	Este Ejercicio de Abrir y Cerrar los Labios le ayuda a aumentar la fuerza, tono, y movimiento de sus labios. Este ejercicio puede ayudarle a evitar que la comida o líquido se tire de su boca.
	Instruction in English	**Instrucción en Español**
Clinician	1. Please open your mouth as wide as you can. 2. Please close your lips and hold them together as tight as you can for 3 seconds. 3. Please repeat this exercise 10 times.	1. Por favor abra su boca lo más ancho que pueda. 2. Por favor cierre sus labios y deténgalos juntos lo más apretados que pueda por 3 segundos. 3. Por favor repita este ejercicio 10 veces.

Treatment for Oral Preparatory Phase Disorders
Strengthening the Lips
Protocol 3.15 (English/Spanish)

Pucker and Smile Exercise

The *Pucker and Smile Exercise* is a set of procedures used to increase lip closure, to decrease spillage of liquid and food outside of the oral cavity (Logemann, 1998).

General Procedures
- Instruct the patient to pucker the lips as firmly as possible.
- Have the patient hold the pucker position for 3 seconds.
- Tell the patient to relax and smile as wide as possible.
- Repeat this exercise 10 times or as tolerated.

Potential Benefits of This Exercise
- Increased lip strength
- Increased lip tone

Protocols for Pucker and Smile Exercise: *Explanation and Instruction to the Patient*		
	Explanation in English	**Explicación en Español**
Clinician	The Pucker and Smile Exercise helps to increase the strength and tone in your lips. This exercise may help prevent food or liquid from falling outside of your mouth.	Este Ejercicio de Fruncir y Sonreír le ayuda a aumentar la fuerza y tono de sus labios. Este ejercicio puede ayudarle a evitar que la comida o el líquido se tire de su boca.
	Instruction in English	**Instrucción en Español**
Clinician	1. Please pucker your lips like this [the clinician should model the correct positioning of the lips]. 2. Please hold your lips together for 3 seconds. 3. Please relax your lips and smile as wide as possible. 4. Please hold your smile as wide as you can for 3 seconds. 5. Please repeat this exercise 10 times.	1. Por favor arrugue sus labios así [debe de modelar la posición correcta de los labios]. 2. Por favor retenga sus labios arrugados/fruncidos por 3 segundos. 3. Por favor descanse sus labios y sonríase lo más ancho que pueda. 4. Por favor detenga la sonrisa lo más ancho que pueda por 3 segundos. 5. Por favor haga este ejercicio 10 veces.

Treatment for Oral Preparatory Phase Disorders
Strengthening the Lips
Protocol 3.16 (English/Spanish)

Tight Lip Exercise

The *Tight Lip Exercise* is a set of procedures used to increase lip closure to decrease spillage of liquid and food outside of the oral cavity (Boshart, 1998; Gangale, 1993; Murry & Carrau, 2006).

General Procedures

- Use a straw, twist-tie, or even a piece of tissue.
- Instruct the patient to place the straw, twist-tie, or piece of tissue between the lips and close the lips tightly.
- Tell the patient to keep a firm lip seal for at least 10 seconds.
- Repeat this exercise 10 times or as tolerated.

Potential Benefits of This Exercise

- Increased lip strength
- Increased sensory awareness
- Increased cheek strength
- Increased lip closure
- Decreased drooling

Protocols for Tight Lip Exercise: *Explanation and Instruction to the Patient*		
	Explanation in English	**Explicación en Español**
Clinician	The Tight Lip Exercise helps you increase the strength and tone in your lips. This exercise may help you to keep the food and liquid from spilling out of your mouth.	Este Ejercicio de El Labio Apretado le ayuda a aumentar la fuerza y tono de sus labios. Este ejercicio puede ayudarle a guardar que la comida o el líquido no se tiren de la boca.
	Instruction in English	**Instrucción en Español**
Clinician	1. I will give you a tissue/straw/twist-tie and I want you to place it between your lips. 2. Please close your lips as tightly as possible so that the object does not fall out of your mouth. 3. Please hold the twist-tie straw/tissue for 10 seconds. 4. Please repeat this exercise 10 times.	1. Voy a darle un papel/popote/alambre y quiero que se lo ponga entre sus labios. 2. Por favor cierre sus labios lo más apretado que pueda para que el objeto no se caiga de su boca. 3. Quiero que retenga el alambre/popote/papel por 10 segundos. 4. Por favor repita este ejercicio 10 veces.

Treatment for Oral Preparatory Phase Disorders
Strengthening the Lips
Protocol 3.17 (English/Spanish)

Big Smile Exercise

The *Big Smile Exercise* is a set of procedures used to increase lip closure, to decrease spillage of food or liquid outside of the oral cavity (O'Sullivan, Godfrey, Van Boldrick, & Puntil, 1990).

General Procedures
- Use a mirror during the treatment session (to increase symmetrical pulling of the lips).
- Have the patient smile as big and wide as possible without showing the teeth.
- Instruct the patient to smile for 3 seconds and then relax the lips.
- Repeat this exercise 10 times or as tolerated.

Potential Benefits of This Exercise
- Increased lip strength
- Increased lip tone
- Increased lip range of motion
- Increased cheek strength
- Increased cheek tone

Protocols for Big Smile Exercise: *Explanation and Instruction to the Patient*		
	Explanation in English	**Explicación en Español**
Clinician	The Big Smile Exercise helps you increase the strength, tone, and movement of your lips.	Este Ejercicio de Sonrisa Grande le ayuda a aumentar la fuerza, tono, y movimiento de sus labios.
	Instruction in English	**Instrucción en Español**
Clinician	1. Please smile as big and wide as you can, without showing your teeth.	1. Por favor sonríase lo más grande y ancho que pueda, sin enseñar sus dientes.
	2. Please hold your smile for 3 seconds.	2. Por favor retenga su sonrisa por 3 segundos.
	3. Please relax your lips.	3. Por favor descanse sus labios.
	4. Please repeat this exercise 10 times.	4. Por favor repita este ejercicio 10 veces.

Treatment for Oral Preparatory Phase Disorders
Strengthening the Cheeks
Protocol 3.18 (English/Spanish)

Cheek Puff Exercise

The *Cheek Puff Exercise* is a set of procedures used to increase lip closure to decrease spillage of food or liquid outside of the oral cavity (Gangale, 1993).

General Procedures
- Instruct the patient to close the mouth and puff air into the cheeks.
- Tell the patient to hold the air in the mouth for 3 seconds.
- Repeat this exercise 10 times.

Potential Benefits of This Exercise
- Increased lip strength
- Increased lip tone
- Increased lip rage of motion
- Increased cheek strength
- Increased cheek tone
- Decreased drooling

Protocols for Cheek Puff Exercise: *Explanation and Instruction to the Patient*		
	Explanation in English	**Explicación en Español**
Clinician	The Cheek Puff Exercise helps your cheeks and lips become stronger so that food and liquid does not fall out of your mouth.	Este Ejercicio de Soplo de Mejilla le ayuda a aumentar la fuerza en sus mejillas y labios para que la comida o el líquido no se caiga de su boca.
	Instruction in English	**Instrucción en Español**
Clinician	1. Please close your lips. 2. Please blow air into your cheeks, while keeping your lips closed. 3. Please hold the air in your cheeks for 3 seconds and then let the air go. 4. Please repeat this exercise five times.	1. Por favor cierre sus labios. 2. Por favor sople aire en sus mejillas, mientras que retiene sus labios cerrados. 3. Por favor retenga el aire en sus mejillas por 3 segundos y luego deje salir el aire. 4. Por favor repita este ejercicio 5 veces.

Treatment for Oral Preparatory Phase Disorders
Improving Cheek Tension

Overview

Many patients with oral preparatory phase dysphagia may exhibit pocketing of food in the cheeks. This may be secondary to reduced muscle tension in the cheeks. The strength in the cheeks is important for the following reasons: (a) closing off the lateral sulci between the lower gums and cheeks. (b) preventing food from pocketing inside the cheek, and (c) keeping the food on the tongue so the patient can chew it adequately (Boshart, 1998; Gangale, 1993; Logemann, 1998; Singh, Brockbank, Frost & Tyler, 1995; Swigert, 2000).

Protocols are provided for the following compensatory swallow therapy exercises and rehabilitative swallow therapy technique that may be helpful in improving the cheek tension:

Compensatory Swallow Therapy Exercises

- Cheek Push-up Exercise
- "Oh" Lips Exercise
- Side Pucker Exercise

Rehabilitative Swallow Therapy Technique

- Head Tilt Strategy

Treatment for Oral Preparatory Phase Disorders
Improving Cheek Tension
Protocol 3.19 (English/Spanish)

Cheek Push-up Exercise

The *Cheek Push-up Exercise* is a set of procedures used to increase tension in the cheeks, to decrease pocketing of food (Boshart, 1998; Gangale, 1993; Swigert, 2000).

General Procedures
- Make sure the patient wears gloves when doing this exercise.
- Instruct the patient to place a finger into the center of the right cheek on the side of the teeth. The patient should bite down with the teeth (with the finger placed on the side of the teeth, where it cannot be inadvertently bitten).
- Tell the patient to push the right cheek outward with the finger. The patient completes this exercise 10 times.
- The patient repeats this exercise on the cheek on the left side.

Potential Benefits of This Exercise
- Increased tension in the cheeks
- Increased strength in the cheeks
- Decreased pocketing

Protocols for Cheek Push-up Exercise: *Explanation and Instruction to the Patient*		
	Explanation in English	**Explicación en Español**
Clinician	The Cheek Push-up Exercise helps you to increase the strength and tension in your cheeks.	Este Ejercicio de Levantar la Mejilla le ayuda a aumentar la fuerza y tensión en sus mejillas.
	Instruction in English	**Instrucción en Español**
Clinician	1. Please take your finger and put it inside your right cheek. 2. Please close your teeth together with your finger placed on the side of the closed teeth against the cheek. 3. Please pull your right cheek outward and tense your cheek muscles against your finger. 4. Please repeat this exercise 10 times on the right side. 5. Please repeat this exercise on the left side. 6. Please take your finger and put it inside your left cheek. 7. Please close your teeth together and place your finger on the side of the closed teeth against the cheek. 8. Please pull your left cheek outward and tense your cheek muscles against your finger. 9. Please repeat this exercise 10 times.	1. Por favor tome su dedo y póngaselo adentro de la mejilla derecha. 2. Por favor cierre sus dientes con su dedo puesto al lado de los dientes cerrados contra la mejilla. 3. Por favor estire su mejilla derecha para afuera y tense los músculos de su mejilla contra su dedo. 4. Por favor haga este ejercicio 10 veces en el lado derecho. 5. Por favor repita este ejercicio 10 veces en el lado izquierdo. 6. Por favor tome su dedo y póngaselo adentro de la mejilla izquierda. 7. Por favor cierre sus dientes con su dedo puesto al lado de los dientes cerrados contra la mejilla. 8. Por favor estire su mejilla izquierda para afuera y tense la mejilla contra su dedo. 9. Por favor repita este ejercicio 10 veces.

Treatment for Oral Preparatory Phase Disorders
Improving Cheek Tension
Protocol 3.20 (English/Spanish)

"Oh" Lips Exercise

The *"Oh" Lips Exercise* is a set of procedures used to increase tension in the cheeks, to reduce pocketing of food (O'Sullivan, Godfrey, Van Boldrik, & Puntil, 1990).

General Procedures
- Utilize a mirror to focus on symmetry and tension needed for lip rounding.
- Instruct the patient to round the lips and say "oh."
- Have the patient hold the production for 5 seconds.
- Repeat this exercise 10 times.

Potential Benefits of This Exercise
- Increased lip strength
- Increased cheek strength
- Increased cheek tension
- Decreased pocketing

Protocols for "Oh" Lips Exercise: *Explanation and Instruction to the Patient*		
	Explanation in English	**Explicación en Español**
Clinician	The "Oh" Lips Exercise helps you increase the strength and tension in your cheeks. This exercise may help you to keep food from sticking inside your cheek.	Este Ejercicio de "O" de Labios le ayuda a aumentar la fuerza y tensión en sus mejillas. Este ejercicio le puede ayudar a asegurar que la comida no se quede en sus mejillas.
	Instruction in English	**Instrucción en Español**
Clinician	1. Please say "Oh" and round your lips as tight as you can. 2. Please keep saying "Oh" for 5 seconds. 3. Please repeat this exercise 10 times.	1. Por favor diga "O" y redondee sus labios lo más apretado que pueda. 2. Por favor siga diciendo "O" por 5 segundos. 3. Por favor repita este ejercicio 10 veces.

Treatment for Oral Preparatory Phase Disorders
Improving Cheek Tension
Protocol 3.21 (English/Spanish)

Side Pucker Exercise

The *Side Pucker Exercise* is a set of procedures used to increase tension in the cheeks that reduces pocketing of food in the oral cavity (Boshart, 1998; Gangale, 1993).

General Procedures

- Use a mirror to increase cheek symmetry and visual feedback for the patient.
- Instruct the patient to pucker and pull the lips completely to the left side and then to the right side.
- Tell the patient to hold the lips in this position on each side for 1 to 3 seconds.
- Repeat this exercise 10 times.

Potential Benefits of This Exercise

- Increased cheek strength
- Increased cheek tension
- Increased lip strength
- Increased lip tension
- Decreased pocketing

Protocols for Side Pucker Exercise: *Explanation and Instruction to the Patient*		
	Explanation in English	**Explicación en Español**
Clinician	The Side Pucker Exercise helps you to increase the tension in your lips and cheeks. This exercise may help you to keep food out of the inside of your cheek.	Este Ejercicio de El Lado Fruncido el Lado le ayuda aumentar la tensión en sus labios y mejillas. Este ejercicio le puede ayudar a prevenir que la comida no se meta adentro de las mejillas.
	Instruction in English	**Instrucción en Español**
Clinician	1. Please pucker your lips and move your lips to the right side. 2. Please hold your lips in that position for 3 seconds. 3. Please repeat this exercise 10 times. 4. Please repeat this exercise on the left side. 5. Please pucker your lips and move your lips to the left side. 6. Please hold your lips in that position for 3 seconds. 7. Please repeat this exercise 10 times.	1. Por favor frunza los labios y muévalos al lado derecho. 2. Por favor detenga sus labios en esta posición 3 segundos. 3. Por favor repita este ejercicio 10 veces. 4. Por favor repita este ejercicio con el lado izquierdo. 5. Por favor frunza sus labios y muévalos al lado izquierdo. 6. Por favor detenga sus labios en esta posición por 3 segundos. 7. Quiero que repita este ejercicio 10 veces.

Treatment for Oral Preparatory Phase Disorders
Improving Cheek Tension
Protocol 3.22 (English/Spanish)

Head Tilt Strategy

The *Head Tilt Strategy* is a set of procedures used to compensate for decreased tension in the patient's cheeks (Buckley, Addicks, & Maniglia, 1976; Logemann, 1998; Singh, Brockbank, Frost, & Tyler, 1995; Swigert, 2000).

General Procedures
- Make sure the patient is on the safest possible oral diet before implementing this compensatory strategy and is not at risk for aspiration.
- Instruct the patient to tilt the head toward the unaffected side while eating food.
- Repeat this strategy during mealtimes.

Potential Benefits of This Strategy
- Increased chewing ability
- Decreased pocketing of food or liquid

Protocols for Head Tilt Strategy: *Explanation and Instruction to the Patient*		
	Explanation in English	**Explicación en Español**
Clinician	The Head Tilt Strategy helps to make sure that food or liquid does not get stuck in the side of your cheek.	Esta Estrategia de Inclinar la Cabeza le ayuda asegurar que la comida o líquido no se pegue en el lado de su mejilla.
	Instruction in English	**Instrucción en Español**
Clinician	1. Please tilt your head toward the right side/left side [whichever side of the tongue is the stronger] while you are eating and swallowing. 2. Please use this strategy whenever you put food into your mouth.	1. Por favor incline su cabeza al lado derecho/izquierdo [segun el lado más fuerte de la lengua] mientras que coma y trague. 2. Por favor use esta estrategia cada vez que se pone comida en la boca.

Treatment for Oral Preparatory Phase Disorders
Improving Tongue Movements

Overview

Patients who exhibit oral preparatory phase dysphagia may have difficulty moving the tongue laterally. The lateral movement of the tongue is important for (a) placing food onto the teeth for mastication, (b) moving the food or liquid from side-to-side with the tongue, and (c) moving oral residue in the cheeks. Both compensatory swallow therapy exercises and rehabilitative swallow therapy strategies may be used for patients who exhibit decreased lateral tongue movement.

Compensatory Swallow Therapy Exercises

Protocols are provided for the following compensatory swallow therapy exercises to improve lateral tongue movement (Gangale, 1993; Logemann, 1998; Murry & Carrau, 2006; Swigert, 2000):

- Side-to-Side Tongue Wag Exercise
- Side Tongue Hold Exercise
- Teeth Sweep Exercise
- Tongue-to-Cheek Push Exercise
- Lateral Tongue Push Exercise
- Lateral Lick Exercise
- Lateral Chew Exercise

Rehabilitative Swallow Therapy Strategies

Protocols are provided for the following rehabilitative swallow therapy strategies (Buckley, Addicks, & Maniglia,1976; Logemann, 1998; Murry & Carrau, 2006; Singh, Brockbank, Frost, & Tyler, 1995):

- Tongue Press Exercise/Strategy
- Head Tilt Strategy

Treatment for Oral Preparatory Phase Disorders
Improving Tongue Movements
Protocol 3.23 (English/Spanish)

Side-to-Side Tongue Wag Exercise

The *Side-to-Side Tongue Wag Exercise* is a set of procedures used to increase lateral tongue movement (Murry & Carrau, 2006).

General Procedures
- Instruct the patient to stick out the tongue and move it from the left to the right side.
- Repeat this exercise 10 times.
- Then have the patient move the tongue from the right side to the left side.

Potential Benefits of This Exercise
- Decreased risk of food falling into the airway
- Increased chewing skills
- Increased strength of the tongue
- Increased range of motion in the tongue

Protocols for Side-to-Side Tongue Wag Exercise: *Explanation and Instruction to the Patient*		
	Explanation in English	**Explicación en Español**
Clinician	The Side-to-Side Tongue Wag Exercise helps you to increase the movement of your tongue from side to side. This exercise may help you move the food in your mouth from one side to the other side.	Este Ejercicio de Meneo de Lengua le ayuda a aumentar el movimiento de lado a lado de su lengua. Este ejercicio puede ayudarle a mover la comida de lado a lado.
	Instruction in English	**Instrucción en Español**
Clinician	1. Please stick out your tongue as far as you can. 2. Please move your tongue from the left side of your mouth to the right side of your mouth as fast as you can. 3. Please repeat this exercise 10 times. 4. Please stick out your tongue as far as you can. 5. Please move your tongue from the right side of your mouth to the left side of your mouth as fast as you can. 6. Please repeat this exercise 10 times.	1. Por favor saque la lengua para afuera todo lo que se pueda. 2. Por favor mueva su lengua de lado a lado lo más rápido que pueda. 3. Por favor repita este ejercicio 10 veces. 4. Por favor saque su lengua todo lo que pueda. 5. Por favor mueva su lengua del lado derecho de su boca al lado izquierdo de su boca lo más rápido que pueda. 6. Por favor repita este ejercicio 10 veces.

Treatment for Oral Preparatory Phase Disorders
Improving Tongue Movements
Protocol 3.24 (English/Spanish)

Side Tongue Hold Exercise

The *Side Tongue Hold Exercise* is a set of procedures used to increase lateral tongue movement (Logemann, 1998).

General Procedures
- Use a mirror throughout the treatment session.
- Tell the patient to stick out the tongue and then move the tongue to the right side.
- Instruct the patient to hold the tongue to the right side for 5 seconds.
- Instruct the patient to relax.
- Repeat this exercise to the left side, with the tongue held in position for 5 seconds.
- Repeat this exercise 10 times.

Potential Benefits of This Exercise
- Increased tongue strength
- Increased range of movement in the tongue
- Increased chewing skills
- Decreased choking risk

Protocols for Side Tongue Hold Exercise: *Explanation and Instruction to the Patient*		
	Explanation in English	**Explicación en Español**
Clinician	The Side Tongue Hold Exercise helps you increase the strength and movement in your tongue. This exercise may help you to chew your food adequately.	Este Ejercicio de Sostener el Lado de la Lengua le ayuda a aumentar la fuerza y movimiento en su lengua. Este ejercicio puede ayudarle a masticar su comida adecuadamente.
	Instruction in English	**Instrucción en Español**
Clinician	1. Please stick out your tongue. 2. Please move your tongue to the right side. 3. Please hold your tongue in that position for 5 seconds. 4. Please relax. 5. Please move your tongue to the left side of your mouth. 6. Please hold your tongue on the left side of your mouth for 5 seconds. 7. I want you to repeat this exercise 10 times.	1. Por favor saque su lengua. 2. Por favor mueva su lengua para el lado derecho. 3. Por favor retenga su lengua en esta posición por 5 segundos. 4. Ahora descanse. 5. Por favor mueva su lengua para el lado izquierdo de su boca. 6. Por favor retenga su lengua en el lado izquierdo de su boca por 5 minutos. 7. Por favor repita este ejercicio 10 veces.

Treatment for Oral Preparatory Phase Disorders
Improving Tongue Movements
Protocol 3.25 (English/Spanish)

Teeth Sweep Exercise

The *Teeth Sweep Exercise* is a set of procedures used to increase lateral tongue movement (Gangale, 1993).

General Procedures
- Have the patient move the tongue against the outside surface of the upper teeth.
- Instruct the patient to slide the tongue (keeping in contact with the upper teeth) all the way to the right side as far as the tongue will go.
- Instruct the patient to hold the tongue to the right side for 5 seconds.
- Repeat this exercise, moving the tongue along the outside surface of the upper teeth to the left side.
- Repeat this exercise 10 times.

Potential Benefits of This Exercise
- Increased range of the tongue
- Increased strength of the tongue
- Increased chewing skills
- Decreased risk for choking

Protocols for Teeth Sweep Exercise: *Explanation and Instruction to the Patient*		
	Explanation in English	**Explicación en Español**
Clinician	The Teeth Sweep Exercise helps you to increase the strength and movement of your tongue so that you can chew your food adequately.	Este Ejercicio de Limpiar los Dientes le ayuda a aumentar la fuerza y movimiento de su lengua para que mastique su comida adecuadamente.
	Instruction in English	**Instrucción en Español**
Clinician	1. Please place the tip of your tongue up against the upper teeth. 2. Next, please slide your tongue against the upper teeth toward the right side all the way to the upper back teeth in your mouth. 3. Please hold your tongue in this position for 5 seconds. 4. Please repeat this exercise 10 times. 5. Please place the tip of your tongue up against the upper teeth. 6. Next, please slide your tongue against the upper teeth toward the left side all the way to the upper back teeth in your mouth. 7. Please hold your tongue in this position for 5 seconds. 8. Please repeat this exercise 10 times.	1. Por favor ponga la punta de su lengua hacia arriba contra los dientes de arriba. 2. Por favor resbale su lengua contra los dientes de arriba hacia el lado derecho todo el camino hasta que llegue a los dientes de atrás. 3. Por favor retenga su lengua en esta posición por 5 minutos. 4. Por favor repita estos ejercicios 10 veces. 5. Por favor ponga la punta de su lengua hacia arriba contra los dientes de arriba. 6. Por favor resbale su lengua contra los dientes de arriba hacia el lado izquierdo hasta que llegue a los dientes de atrás dc su boca. 7. Por favor retenga su lengua en esta posición por 5 segundos. 8. Por favor repita este ejercicio 10 veces.

Treatment for Oral Preparatory Phase Disorders
Improving Tongue Movements
Protocol 3.26 (English/Spanish)

Tongue-to-Cheek Push Exercise

The *Tongue-to-Cheek Push Exercise* is a set of procedures used to increase lateral movement of the tongue (Swigert, 2000).

General Procedures
- Instruct the patient to move the tongue toward the right inner side of the cheek.
- Place a gloved finger on the patient's external cheek.
- Have the patient use their tongue to push their cheek against the clinician's gloved finger.
- Instruct the patient to continue pushing the tongue against the clinician's finger for 5 seconds or as long as the patient can tolerate.
- Have the patient place the tongue inside the left inner cheek.
- Repeat this exercise 10 times.

Potential Benefits of This Exercise
- Increased strength of the tongue
- Increased range of the tongue
- Increased chewing skills
- Decreased risk for choking

Protocols for Tongue-to-Cheek Push Exercise: *Explanation and Instruction to the Patient*		
	Explanation in English	**Explicación en Español**
Clinician	The Tongue-to-Cheek Push Exercise helps you increase the strength and movement of your tongue. This exercise may help you chew your food adequately.	Este Ejercicio de Empujón de Lengua a Mejilla le ayuda a aumentar la fuerza y movimiento de su lengua. Este ejercicio puede ayudarle a masticar su comida adecuadamente.
	Instruction in English	**Instrucción en Español**
Clinician	1. Please move your tongue and place it inside the inner cheek on your right side.	1. Por favor mueva su lengua y póngala adentro de la mejilla derecha.
	2. I will place my finger against your cheek on the outside.	2. Voy a poner mi dedo contra su mejilla por afuera.
	3. Please push your cheek against my finger with your tongue as hard as you can and keep pushing for 5 seconds.	3. Por favor empuje su mejilla contra mi dedo con su lengua lo más fuerte que pueda y siga empujando por 5 segundos.
	4. Please repeat this exercise 10 times.	4. Por favor repita este ejercicio 10 veces.
	5. Please move your tongue and place it inside the inner cheek on your left side.	5. Por favor mueva su lengua póngala adentro de la mejilla izquierda.
	6. I will place my finger against the outside of your cheek.	6. Voy a poner mi dedo contra su mejilla por afuera.
	7. Please push your cheek against my finger with your tongue as hard as you can and keep pushing for 5 seconds.	7. Por favor empuje su mejilla contra mi dedo con su lengua lo más fuerte que pueda y siga empujando por 5 segundos.
	8. Please repeat this exercise 10 times.	8. Por favor repita este ejercicio 10 veces.

Treatment for Oral Preparatory Phase Disorders
Improving Tongue Movements
Protocol 3.27 (English/Spanish)

Lateral Tongue Push Exercise

The *Lateral Tongue Push Exercise* is a set of procedures used to increase lateral movement of the tongue (Swigert, 2000).

General Procedures
- Use a mirror throughout this treatment exercise.
- Have a tongue depressor available.
- Instruct the patient to stick out the tongue to the right side of the mouth.
- Place the flat side of the tongue depressor on the right side of the patient's tongue.
- Instruct the patient to push the tongue against the tongue depressor as hard as possible.
- Instruct the patient to push against the tongue depressor for 5 seconds.
- Repeat this exercise on the left side of the tongue.
- Complete 10 trials of this exercise, or as many trials as the patient can tolerate.

Potential Benefits of This Exercise
- Increased muscle tone
- Increased muscle strength
- Increased lateral movement of the tongue
- Increased formation of an adequate bolus

Protocols for Lateral Tongue Push Exercise: *Explanation and Instruction to the Patient*		
	Explanation in English	**Explicación en Español**
Clinician	The Lateral Tongue Push Exercise helps you move your food, with your tongue, from one side of your mouth to the other side. This exercise may help you chew your food better.	Este Ejercicio de Empujón de los Lados de la Lengua le ayuda a mover su comida, con su lengua, de un lado de la boca al otro. Este ejercicio puede ayudarle a masticar su comida mejor.
	Instruction in English	**Instrucción en Español**
Clinician	1. Please open your mouth and stick out your tongue. 2. I will place a tongue depressor to the right side of your face. 3. Please stretch your tongue out and press it against the tongue depressor as hard as you can. 4. Please press your tongue against the tongue depressor for 5 seconds. 5. Please repeat this exercise 10 times. 6. Please open your mouth and stick out your tongue. 7. I will place a tongue depressor to the left side of your face. 8. Please stretch your tongue out and press it against the tongue depressor as hard as you can. 9. Please press against the tongue depressor for 5 seconds. 10. Please repeat this exercise 10 times.	1. Por favor abra su boca y saque su lengua. 2. Voy a ponerle un depresor de la lengua al lado derecho de su cara. 3. Por favor estire su lengua para afuera y aplánela contra el depresor lo más fuerte que pueda. 4. Por favor apriete su lengua contra el depresor por 5 segundos. 5. Por favor repita este ejercicio 10 veces. 6. Por favor abra su boca y saque su lengua. 7. Voy a ponerle un depresor de la lengua al lado izquierda de su cara. 8. Por favor estire su lengua para afuera y aplánela contra el depresor lo más fuerte que pueda. 9. Por favor aprieté su lengua contra el depresor por 5 segundos. 10. Por favor repita este ejercicio 10 veces.

Treatment for Oral Preparatory Phase Disorders
Improving Tongue Movements
Protocol 3.28 (English/Spanish)

Lateral Lick Exercise

The *Lateral Lick Exercise* is a set of procedures used to increase lateral movement of the tongue (Logemann, 1998).

General Procedures
- Make sure that the patient is at a stage in therapy that is safe for consumption of food without the risk of aspiration or choking.
- Make sure that the patient is not allergic to peanut butter.
- Check the patient's diet for special considerations when presenting oral trials of food (e.g., diabetic or low-salt diet).
- Put a minimal amount of peanut butter or applesauce on the tongue depressor (e.g., enough applesauce or peanut butter to coat the tip of the tongue depressor on one side).
- Put peanut butter or applesauce on the tip of a tongue depressor.
- Place the tongue depressor toward the outer right side of the patient's tongue.
- Instruct the patient to stick out the tongue toward the right side and lick the peanut butter or applesauce off of the tongue depressor.
- Repeat 10 trials of this exercise.
- Alternate this exercise to the left side of the tongue.

Potential Benefits of This Exercise
- Increased range of motion of the tongue
- Increased strength of the tongue
- Increased sensory awareness of the tongue
- Increased chewing skills

Protocols for Lateral Lick Exercise: *Explanation and Instruction to the Patient*		
	Explanation in English	**Explicación en Español**
Clinician	The Lateral Lick Exercise helps you to strengthen your tongue. This exercise may help you chew and move the food in your mouth from one side to the other side.	Este ejercicio le ayuda a fortalecer su lengua. Este ejercicio le puede ayudar a masticar y mover la comida en su boca de un lado al otro.
	Instruction in English	**Instrucción en Español**
Clinician	1. I will put a tongue depressor with applesauce next to your mouth on the right side. 2. Please stick out your tongue to the right side of your mouth and lick the apple sauce off the tongue depressor. 3. Please repeat this exercise 10 times. 4. I will place a tongue depressor with applesauce next to your mouth on the left side. 5. Please stick out your tongue to the left side of your mouth and lick the applesauce off the tongue depressor. 6. Please repeat this exercise 10 times.	1. Voy a poner un depresor de lengua con puré de manzana enseguida de su boca al lado derecho. 2. Por favor saque su lengua al lado derecho y lamba el puré de manzana del depresor. 3. Por favor repita este ejercicio 10 veces. 4. Voy a ponerle un depresor de lengua con puré de manzana enseguida de su boca al lado izquierdo. 5. Por favor saque su legua al lado izquierdo y lamba el puré de manzana del depresor. 6. Por favor repita este ejercicio 10 veces.

Treatment for Oral Preparatory Phase Disorders
Improving Tongue Movements
Protocol 3.29 (English/Spanish)

Lateral Chew Exercise

The *Lateral Chew Exercise* is a set of procedures used to increase lateral movement of the tongue (Gangale, 1993; Logemann, 1998, Murry & Carrau, 2006).

General Procedures
- Prepare a 5-inch by 5-inch piece of gauze.
- Have the patient open the mouth.
- Place the gauze strip at the midline on the patient's tongue.
- Hold one side of the gauze strip while the patient is chewing on the other side of the gauze strip.
- Instruct the patient to move the gauze strip with the tongue to the right side of the mouth.
- Have the patient chew the gauze strip five times on the right side of the mouth.
- Instruct the patient to move the gauze strip with the tongue to the left side of the mouth.
- Have the patient chew the gauze strip five times on the left side of the mouth.
- Have the patient repeat this exercise 10 times.

Potential Benefits of This Exercise
- Increased lateral movement of the tongue
- Increased tongue strength
- Increased chewing skills
- Increased bolus formation

Protocols for Lateral Chew Exercise: *Explanation and Instruction to the Patient*		
	Explanation in English	**Explicación en Español**
Clinician	The Lateral Chew Exercise helps you to push the food in your mouth from side to side.	Este Ejercicio del Masticado Lateral le ayuda a empujar la comida en su boca de un lado al otro.
	Instruction in English	**Instrucción en Español**
Clinician	1. I will put a piece of gauze in your mouth and place it on the middle of your tongue. 2. I will hold onto one side of the gauze. 3. Please move the gauze with your tongue to the left side and chew five times. 4. Please move the gauze from the left side of your mouth to the right side and chew five times. 5. Please repeat this exercise 10 times.	1. Voy a poner un pedazo de gasa en su boca se la voy a poner en medio de la lengua. 2. Yo detengo un lado de la gasa. 3. Por favor mueva la gasa con su lengua al lado izquierdo y mastique 5 veces. 4. Por favor mueva la gasa del lado izquierdo de su boca al lado derecho y mastique 5 veces. 5. Por favor repita este ejercicio 10 veces.

Treatment for Oral Preparatory Phase Disorders
Improving Tongue Movements
Protocol 3.30 (English/Spanish)

Tongue Press Exercise/Strategy

The *Tongue Press Exercise/Strategy* is a set of procedures used for patients that exhibit decreased lateral movement of the tongue (Logemann, 1998; Buckley, Addicks, & Maniglia, 1976, Murry & Carrau, 2006).

General Procedures
- Implement this exercise/strategy only for patients who exhibit adequate tongue elevation up to the hard palate.
- Train the patient to press the tongue against the hard palate. At the beginning, the clinician should not incorporate food into this strategy.
- As the patient progresses, introduce food with this strategy.
- The patient repeats this exercise/strategy 10 times, or as tolerated.

Potential Benefits of This Exercise/Strategy
- Increased ability to chew food adequately
- Decreased risk of choking on food

Protocols for Tongue Press Exercise/Strategy: *Explanation and Instruction to the Patient*		
	Explanation in English	**Explicación en Español**
Clinician	The Tongue Press Exercise/Strategy helps you to manage the food in your mouth. This exercise/strategy may help you to move your tongue from side to side.	Este Ejercicio/Estrategia de Apretón de Lengua le ayuda a manejar su comida en su boca. Este ejercicio/estrategia le puede ayudar a mover su lengua de un lado a otro.
	Instruction in English	**Instrucción en Español**
Clinician	1. I will place food on your tongue. 2. Please take the food that I place on your tongue, chew it and move it up to the roof of your mouth. 3. Please mash the food in your mouth by pressing your tongue against the roof of your mouth. 4. Please continue doing this exercise/ strategy whenever you eat a meal.	1. Voy a ponerle comida en su lengua. 2. Por favor tome la comida que le puse en la lengua, mastiquela y muévala hacia el paladar. 3. Por favor machuque la comida en su boca con su lengua apretándola contra el paladar. 4. Por favor siga haciendo este ejercicio/estrategia cuando coma comida.

Treatment for Oral Preparatory Phase Disorders
Improving Tongue Movements
Protocol 3.31 (English/Spanish)

Head Tilt Strategy

The *Head Tilt Strategy* is a set of procedures used with patients who exhibit reduced lateral movement of the tongue (Buckley, Addicks, & Maniglia, 1976; Logemann, 1998; Singh, Brockbank, Frost, & Tyler, 1995).

General Procedures
- Place the food into the patient's mouth.
- Instruct the patient move the head toward the side that is able to maintain adequate control of the bolus.
- Repeat this strategy throughout meals.

Potential Benefits of This Exercise
- Increased ability to chew food adequately
- Decreased choking risks
- Decreased pocketing

Protocols for Head Tilt Strategy: *Explanation and Instruction to the Patient*		
	Explanation in English	**Explicación en Español**
Clinician	The Head Tilt Strategy helps you control the food in your mouth. This strategy may help you chew your food more adequately.	Esta Estrategia de Inclinar la Cabeza le ayuda a controlar la comida en su boca. Esta estrategia le puede ayudar a masticar su comida.
	Instruction in English	**Instrucción en Español**
Clinician	1. I will put some food into your mouth. 2. Please tilt your head to the left/right (whichever side has better control), chew it then swallow. 3. Please continue this strategy while you eat.	1. Voy a ponerle comida en su boca. 2. Por favor incline su cabeza a la izquierda/dcrccha (scgún el lado que tenga mejor control) mastíquela y luego trague. 3. Por favor siga esta estrategia mientras que coma.

Treatment for Oral Preparatory Phase Disorders
Improving Tongue Tip Elevation

Overview

Exercises to Increase Tongue Tip Elevation

Patients with oral preparatory phase dysphagia may not have the strength to move the tongue vertically. Vertical movement of the tongue provides contact between the tongue and the hard palate. Generally, the tip of the tongue and the lateral margins of the tongue are positioned against the alveolar ridge during the swallow (Dodds, Taylor, Stewart, Kern, Logemann, & Cook, 1989).

Protocols are provided for the following compensatory swallow therapy exercises that may be helpful in improving tongue tip elevation (Boshart, 1998; Gangale, 1993; Murry & Carrau, 2006):

Compensatory Swallow Therapy Exercises

- Tongue Tip Push Exercise
- Toothette Squeeze Exercise
- Anterior Tongue Click Exercise
- Tongue Tip Sound Production Exercise
- Tongue Tip Swipe Exercise

Treatment for Oral Preparatory Phase Disorders
Improving Tongue Tip Elevation
Protocol 3.32 (English/Spanish)

Tongue Tip Push Exercise

The *Tongue Tip Push Exercise* is a set of procedures used to increase vertical movement of the tongue (Murry & Carrau, 2006).

General Procedures
- Use a mirror during this exercise to provide visual feedback.
- Have the patient push the tongue tip up against the alveolar ridge.
- Repeat this exercise 10 times.

Potential Benefits of This Exercise
- Increased tongue tip elevation
- Decreased oral transit time
- Decreased tongue thrust swallow

Protocols for Tongue Tip Push Exercise: *Explanation and Instruction to the Patient*		
	Explanation in English	**Explicación en Español**
Clinician	The Tongue Tip Push Exercise helps to increase the strength in your tongue. This exercise may help you hold food in your mouth.	Este Ejercicio de Empujón de la Punta de la Lengua le ayuda a aumentar la fuerza de su lengua. Este ejercicio le puede ayudar a retener la comida en su boca.
	Instruction in English	**Instrucción en Español**
Clinician	1. I will show you where I want you to place your tongue [the clinician takes a tongue depressor and presses on the alveolar ridge]. 2. Please lift the tip of your tongue up and push against the area that I showed you. 3. Please keep your tongue in that position for 3 seconds. 4. Please complete this exercise 10 times.	1. Voy a enseñarle donde quiero que ponga su lengua (la terapista debe de tomar el depresor de lengua y apretar en el proceso alveolar). 2. Por favor levante la punta de la lengua y empuje contra el área que le enseñe. 3. Por favor mantenga su lengua en esta posición por 3 segundos. 4. Por favor haga este ejercicio 10 veces.

Treatment for Oral Preparatory Phase Disorders
Improving Tongue Tip Elevation
Protocol 3.33 (English/Spanish)

Toothette Squeeze Exercise

The *Toothette Squeeze Exercise* is a set of procedures used to increase vertical tongue movement (Boshart, 1998).

General Procedures
- Use a Toothette for this exercise.
- Provide a mirror during this exercise to provide visual feedback.
- Place the Toothette on the patient's alveolar ridge.
- Instruct the patient to push up against the Toothette with the tongue.
- Repeat this exercise 10 times.

Potential Benefits of This Exercise
- Increased tongue tip strength
- Increased tongue tip range
- Decreased tongue thrust swallow

Protocols for Toothette Squeeze Exercise: *Explanation and Instruction to the Patient*		
	Explanation in English	**Explicación en Español**
Clinician	The Toothette Squeeze Exercise helps to increase your tongue strength. This exercise may help you hold food in your mouth.	Este Ejercicio de Apretón con Esponjita le ayuda a aumentar la fuerza de su lengua. Este ejercicio le puede ayudar a retener la comida en su boca.
	Instruction in English	**Instrucción en Español**
Clinician	1. I will place this mirror in front of you so you can see if you are doing this exercise correctly. 2. Please open your mouth. 3. I will place a Toothette behind your upper front teeth. 4. Please move the tip of your tongue up and push against the sponge. 5. Please repeat this exercise 10 times.	1. Voy a poner este espejo frente a usted para que mire si esta haciendo el ejercicio correcto. 2. Por favor abra su boca. 3. Voy a poner una esponjita atrás de sus dientes de arriba. 4. Por favor mueva la punta de la lengua hacia arriba y empuje contra la esponjita. 5. Por favor repita este ejercicio 10 veces.

Treatment for Oral Preparatory Phase Disorders
Improving Tongue Tip Elevation
Protocol 3.34 (English/Spanish)

Anterior Tongue Click Exercise

The *Anterior Tongue Click Exercise* is a set of procedures used to increase vertical tongue movement (Boshart, 1998; Gangale, 1993; Murry & Carrau, 2006).

General Procedures
• Provide a mirror for the patient to provide visual feedback.
• Instruct the patient to click the tip of the tongue against the anterior portion of the palate.
• Repeat 10 trials of this exercise.

Potential Benefits of This Exercise
• Increased tongue tip strength
• Increased tongue tip range
• Increased tongue tip sensory awareness

Protocols for Anterior Tongue Click Exercise: *Explanation and Instruction to the Patient*		
	Explanation in English	**Explicación en Español**
Clinician	The Anterior Tongue Click Exercise helps increase the strength in the tip of your tongue. This exercise may help you to move the food or liquid in your mouth more easily.	Este Ejercicio de Clic Anterior de la Lengua le ayuda a aumentar la fuerza en la punta de su lengua. Este ejercicio le puede ayudar a mover la comida o el líquido en su boca con más facilidad.
	Instruction in English	**Instrucción en Español**
Clinician	1. I will show you where I want you to click the tip of your tongue (the clinician shows the patient with a tongue depressor where to place the tip of the tongue). 2. Please click the tip of your tongue against the spot where I showed you. 3. Please repeat this exercise 10 times.	1. Quiero enseñarle donde quiero que haga clic con la punta de la lengua (la terapista le debe de enseñar al paciente con un depresor de lengua donde debe de poner la punta de la lengua). 2. Por favor haga clic con la punta de su lengua contra el lugar que le enseñe. 3. Por favor repita este ejercicio 10 veces.

Treatment for Oral Preparatory Phase Disorders
Improving Tongue Tip Elevation
Protocol 3.35 (English/Spanish)

Tongue Tip Sound Production Exercise

The *Tongue Tip Sound Production Exercise* is a set of procedures used to increase vertical movement of the tongue (Murry & Carrau, 2006).

General Procedures
- Provide a mirror throughout this exercise to give the patient visual feedback.
- Instruct the patient to say words that contain the /t/, /d/, or /l/ phoneme in the initial position.

Complete a list of words two times.

Potential Benefits of This Exercise
- Increased tongue tip strength
- Increased vertical movement of the tongue
- Increased tongue tip formation that is needed to initiate the swallow

Protocols for Tongue Tip Sound Production Exercise: *Explanation and Instruction to the Patient*		
	Explanation in English	**Explicación en Español**
Clinician	The Tongue Tip Sound Production Exercise helps to increase the strength in the tip of your tongue. This exercise may help you to form the food in your mouth into a ball that is appropriate for you to swallow.	Este Ejercicio de Producción de Sonido con la Punta de la Lengua le ayuda a aumentar la fuerza en la punta de la lengua. Este ejercicio le puede ayudar a formar la comida en su boca en una bola que es adecuada para que usted trague.
	Instruction in English	**Instrucción en Español**
Clinician	1. I will place a mirror in front of you so you can see if you are doing this exercise correctly. 2. I will give you a list of words to say. 3. Please say these words that have the sounds /t/, /d/, and /l/ in them. 4. Please say them slowly at first and then increase your speed. 5. Please say the word list twice.	1. Voy a ponerle un espejo frente a usted para que mire lo que esta haciendo. 2. Le voy a dar una lista de palabras para que diga. 3. Por favor diga estas palabras que tienen sonidos de /t/, /d/, y /l/ en ellas. 4. Por favor diga las palabras despacio y luego aumente la velocidad. 5. Por favor diga la lista de palabras dos veces.

/t/ Word List in English

1. tab	16. tin	31. too
2. tack	17. tire	32. toss
3. tad	18. tent	33. toy
4. tail	19. test	34. type
5. take	20. teeth	35. tango
6. talk	21. toe	36. table
7. tall	22. ton	37. taco
8. tan	23. toast	38. talent
9. tank	24. tie	39. tired
10. tap	25. taste	40. today
11. tar	26. tube	41. towel
12. tea	27. turn	42. tooth
13. tears	28. two	43. touch
14. ted	29. tongue	44. tiny
15. ten	30. tool	45. tuna

/t/ Word List in Spanish

1. tubo	16. tira	31. tipo
2. torre	17. tío	32. tino
3. tango	18. típico	33. tinte
4. toga	19. tiro	34. tinta
5. tarea	20. tiza	35. tímido
6. tepe	21. todo	36. tila
7. tigre	22. toma	37. terrible
8. tala	23. tomo	38. tesar
9. tomo	24. tono	39. tesoro
10. taga	25. toque	40. tiempo
11. tollo	26. torta	41. temer
12. toso	27. total	42. teme
13. talla	28. toser	43. tejar
14. tapa	29. tortilla	44. tarde
15. toma	30. tortita	45. taza

/d/ Word List in English

1. dance	16. dad	31. door
2. dash	17. dark	32. due
3. day	18. disk	33. dunk
4. dear	19. desk	34. dinner
5. dive	20. dot	35. disease
6. dime	21. dug	36. doctor
7. dodge	22. duck	37. dollar
8. dog	23. dump	38. donate
9. dove	24. denim	39. double
10. dust	25. dancer	40. dozen
11. down	26. daisy	41. duet
12. doll	27. daughter	42. deal
13. dice	28. dye	43. dent
14. deer	29. deep	44. dirt
15. den	30. dip	45. doe

/d/ Word List in Spanish

1. dama	16. defecto	31. desposar
2. dandi	17. déficit	32. destino
3. dante	18. dejar	33. día
4. danza	19. delgado	34. dos
5. dar	20. delgada	35. devolver
6. dañar	21. delito	36. diario
7. data	22. delicia	37. deuda
8. dato	23. demora	38. detrás
9. deber	24. diez	39. dentro
10. débil	25. deparar	40. dicha
11. década	26. deporte	41. diente
12. debito	27. deposito	42. dieta
13. decir	28. derecho	43. digno
14. decoro	29. descripción	44. digna
15. dedo	30. desde	45. dios

/l/ Word List in English

1. lad	16. limb	31. lamb
2. lake	17. lip	32. lady
3. lamp	18. live	33. larger
4. lap	19. lobe	34. later
5. lard	20. lodge	35. lawyer
6. last	21. log	36. lazy
7. late	22. lost	37. leader
8. laugh	23. love	38. lemon
9. lion	24. lawn	39. low
10. leap	25. lump	40. liver
11. least	26. lose	41. lobster
12. led	27. loaf	42. logic
13. lie	28. lime	43. listen
14. life	29. lick	44. limit
15. left	30. land	45. laundry

/l/ Word List in Spanish

1. la	16. leche	31. lancha
2. labio	17. lechuga	32. langosta
3. labor	18. leer	33. ladrillo
4. labrar	19. largo	34. lengua
5. ladilla	20. lentes	35. larga
6. lado	21. ley	36. lector
7. lechón	22. lago	37. libra
8. libre	23. lana	38. libro
9. línea	24. lacio	39. líder
10. lámpara	25. limón	40. litro
11. lápiz	26. limpiar	41. lugar
12. lunes	27. lata	42. linda
13. luz	28. lavar	43. lino
14. lazo	29. lista	44. lapicero
15. lección	30. loma	45. laso

Treatment for Oral Preparatory Phase Disorders
Improving Tongue Tip Elevation
Protocol 3.36 (English/Spanish)

Tongue Tip Swipe Exercise

The *Tongue Tip Swipe Exercise* is a set of procedures used to increase vertical movement of the tongue (Murry & Carrau, 2006; Swigert, 2000).

General Procedures

- Provide a mirror throughout this exercise to give the patient visual feedback.
- Use a tongue depressor to show the patient the spot on the alveolar ridge where the tongue tip should contact and areas on the hard and soft palates where the tongue should touch.
- Instruct the patient to put the tip of the tongue against the alveolar ridge and slide the tongue tip back against the hard palate and the soft palate.
- Repeat this exercise 10 times.

Potential Benefits of This Exercise

- Increased the tongue tip strength
- Increased vertical movement of the tongue
- Increased tongue tip formation needed for the initiation of the swallow

Protocols for Tongue Tip Swipe Exercise: *Explanation and Instruction to the Patient*		
	Explanation in English	**Explicación en Español**
Clinician	The Tongue Tip Swipe Exercise helps to increase the strength in your tongue. This exercise may help you to hold the food in your mouth adequately before you swallow.	Este Ejercicio de Limpiar la Punta de la Lengua le ayuda a aumentar la fuerza en su lengua. Este ejercicio le puede ayudar a retener la comida en su boca adecuadamente antes de tragar.
	Instruction in English	**Instrucción en Español**
Clinician	1. Please look in this mirror that I put in front of you throughout this exercise.	1. Por favor mire en este espejo que he puesto frente a usted durante este ejercicio.
	2. I will place a tongue depressor on the roof of your mouth [the clinician places the tongue depressor on the alveolar ridge].	2. Voy a poner un depresor de lengua en su paladar (la terapista debe de poner el depresor en el proceso alveolar).
	3. Please put the tip of your tongue on this spot.	3. Por favor ponga la punta de la lengua aquí.
	4. Next, please slide your tongue backward along the roof of your mouth. Then relax and hold it in that position for 3 seconds.	4. Por favor resbale su lengua hacia atrás sobre el paladar luego descanse y deténgala en esta posición por 3 segundos.
	5. Please slide your tongue tip forward along the roof of your mouth toward the front of your mouth.	5. Por favor resbale su punta de la lengua hacia enfrente sobre el paladar a la parte de enfrente de su boca.
	6. Please repeat this exercise 10 times.	6. Por favor repita este ejercicio 10 veces.

Treatment for Oral Preparatory Phase Disorders Improving Tongue Movement for Bolus Formation

Overview

During the oral preparatory phase, the patient should chew solid food and form a cohesive bolus that is conducive to a smooth swallow. Patients who exhibit oral preparatory phase dysphagia may have difficulty forming an adequate bolus for the following reasons: (a) reduced movement of the tongue, (b) reduced strength of the tongue, and (c) reduced coordination of the tongue (Logemann, 1998; Murry & Carrau, 2006; Swigert, 2000). In essence, a reduced range of movement of the tongue is mainly responsible for difficulties in forming a bolus.

Protocols are provided for the following compensatory swallow therapy techniques, which can be used to increase the range of tongue movement to form a cohesive bolus (Ford, Grotz, Pomerantz, Bruno, & Flannery, 1974; Logemann, 1998; Swigert, 2000):

- Chewing Gum or Licorice Exercise
- Lateral Tongue Push Exercise
- Middle Tongue Push Exercise
- Back Tongue Push-up Exercise

Treatment for Oral Preparatory Phase Disorders
Improving Tongue Movement for Bolus Formation
Protocol 3.37 (English/Spanish)

Chewing Gum or Licorice Exercise

The *Chewing Gum or Licorice Exercise* is a set of procedures used to increase oral sensitivity (Ford, Grotz, Pomerantz, Bruno, & Flannery, 1974; Logemann, 1998).

General Procedures
- Give the patient a small to medium-sized piece of gum or licorice to chew.
- Instruct the patient to chew alternately from the right side to the left side of the mouth.
- Tell the patient not to swallow the gum or licorice.
- Repeat this exercise 10 times.

Note to the Clinician
- Use clinical judgement when deciding to implement this exercise into the patient's therapy program.
- Make sure that the patient is not at risk for aspiration before implementing this strategy.

Potential Benefits of This Exercise
- Increased chewing skills
- Increased sensory awareness of the tongue

Protocol for Chewing Gum or Licorice Exercise: *Explanation and Instruction to the Patient*		
	Explanation in English	**Explanación en Español**
Clinician	The Chewing Gum or Licorice Exercise helps to increase the sensation in your tongue to help you begin your swallow.	Este Ejercicio de Chicle o Regaliz le ayuda a aumentar la sensación en su lengua para ayudarle a comenzar su trago.
	Instruction in English	**Instrucción en Español**
Clinician	1. I will give you a piece of gum or licorice. 2. Please move the gum or licorice in your mouth to the right side and chew. 3. Please move the gum or licorice to your left side and chew. 4. Please repeat this exercise 10 times. 5. Please do not swallow the gum or licorice. 6. Please spit out the gum or licorice onto this napkin. 7. Thank you.	1. Le voy a dar un pedazo de chicle o regaliz. 2. Por favor mueva el chicle o regaliz en su boca al lado derecho y mastique. 3. Por favor mueva el chicle o regaliz al lado izquierdo y mastique. 4. Por favor repita este ejercicio 10 veces. 5. Por favor no se trague el chicle o regaliz. 6. Por favor escupa el chicle o regaliz para afuera en esta servilleta. 7. Gracias.

Treatment for Oral Preparatory Phase Disorders
Improving Tongue Movement for Bolus Formation
Protocol 3.38 (English/Spanish)

Lateral Tongue Push Exercise

The *Lateral Tongue Push Exercise* is a set of procedures used to increase the range of motion of the tongue to form a cohesive bolus (Swigert, 2000).

General Procedures
- Instruct the patient to open the mouth and push the left side of the tongue up against a tongue depressor that the clinician is holding.
- Repeat this exercise 10 times.
- Complete this exercise on the right side of the tongue.

Potential Benefits of This Exercise
- Increased tongue strength
- Increased tongue range
- Increased ability to form a cohesive bolus

Protocols for Lateral Tongue Push Exercise: *Explanation and Instruction to the Patient*		
	Explanation in English	**Explicación en Español**
Clinician	The Lateral Tongue Push Exercise helps to strengthen the sides of your tongue. This exercise may help you to form the food in your mouth into a ball that is adequate for you to swallow.	Este Ejercicio Empujón de los Lados de la Lengua le ayuda a reforzar los lados de su lengua. Este ejercicio le puede ayudar a formar la comida en su boca en un bolo que es adecuado para que usted trague.
	Instruction in English	**Instrucción en Español**
Clinician	1. I will place the tongue depressor on top of the left side of your tongue. 2. Please lift your tongue up against the tongue depressor. 3. Please push your tongue up against the tongue depressor for 5 seconds. 4. Please do this exercise 10 times. 5. Please repeat this exercise on the right side of your tongue. 6. I will place the tongue depressor on top of the right side of your tongue. 7. Please lift your tongue up against the tongue depressor. 8. Please push your tongue up against the tongue depressor for 5 seconds. 9. Please complete this exercise 10 times.	1. Voy a poner un depresor de lengua arriba del lado izquierdo de su lengua. 2. Por favor levante su legua para arriba contra el depresor. 3. Por favor empuje su lengua para arriba contra el depresor por 5 segundos. 4. Por favor haga este ejercicio 10 veces. 5. Por favor repita este ejercicio en el lado derecho de su lengua. 6. Voy a poner un depresor de lengua arriba en el lado derecho de su lengua. 7. Por favor levante su lengua para arriba contra el depresor. 8. Por favor empuje su lengua para arriba contra el depresor por 5 segundos. 9. Por favor haga este ejercicio 10 veces.

Treatment for Oral Preparatory Phase Disorders
Improving Tongue Movement for Bolus Formation
Protocol 3.39 (English/Spanish)

Middle Tongue Push Exercise

The *Middle Tongue Push Exercise* is a set of procedures used to increase the range of motion of the tongue, to support the ability to form a cohesive bolus (Boshart, 1998).

General Procedures
- Use a Toothette sponge.
- Place the Toothette sponge against the hard palate in the patient's oral cavity.
- Instruct the patient to move the middle of the tongue up and push against the Toothette sponge.
- Repeat this exercise 10 times.

Potential Benefits of This Exercise
- Increased strength of the tongue
- Increased range of motion of the tongue to form a cohesive bolus

Protocols for Middle Tongue Push Exercise: *Explanation and Instruction to the Patient*		
	Explanation in English	**Explicación en Español**
Clinician	This Middle Tongue Push Exercise helps to increase the strength in your tongue. This exercise may help you to form the food in your mouth into a ball for you to swallow.	Este Ejercicio de Empujón del Medio de la Lengua le ayuda a aumentar la fuerza en su lengua. Este ejercicio le puede ayudar a formar la comida en su boca en un bolo para que usted trague.
	Instruction in English	**Instrucción en Español**
Clinician	1. I will place the tip of a tongue depressor on the roof of your mouth. 2. Please take the middle of your tongue and press against the spot on the roof of your mouth that I touched. 3. Please press your tongue against the roof of your mouth for 3 seconds. 4. Please repeat this exercise 10 times.	1. Voy a ponerle la punta del depresor en el paladar. 2. Por favor tome la parte del medio de su lengua y aplánela sobre el punto del paladar que he tocado. 3. Por favor aplane su lengua contra el paladar por 3 segundos. 4. Por favor repita este ejercicio 10 veces.

Treatment for Oral Preparatory Phase Disorders
Improving Tongue Movement for Bolus Formation
Protocol 3.40 (English/Spanish)

Back Tongue Push-up Exercise

The *Back Tongue Push-up Exercise* is used to increase the range of motion of the tongue to form a cohesive bolus (Boshart, 1998; Gangale, 1993; Logemann, 1998; Murry & Carrau, 2006; Swigert, 2000).

General Procedures

- Show the patient with a tongue depressor the area of the soft palate where the back of the tongue should contact.
- Instruct the patient to push the back of the tongue up against the soft palate of the oral cavity.
- Instruct the patient to hold this tongue position for 3 seconds.
- Repeat this exercise 10 times.

Potential Benefits of This Exercise

- Increased strength of the back of the tongue
- Increased range of the back of the tongue
- Increased ability to form a bolus

Protocols for Back Tongue Push-up Exercise: *Explanation and Instruction to the Patient*		
	Explanation in English	**Explicación en Español**
Clinician	The Back Tongue Push-up Exercise helps to strengthen the back of your tongue. This exercise may help you form the food in your mouth so that you are able to swallow appropriately.	Este Ejercicio de Levantar la Parte Posterior de la Lengua le ayuda a esforzar la parte posterior de su lengua. Este ejercicio le puede ayudar a formar la comida en su boca para que pueda tragar apropiadamente.
	Instruction in English	**Instrucción en Español**
Clinician	1. Please open your mouth. 2. I will place a tongue depressor in your mouth to show you what area the back of your tongue should touch. 3. Please move the back of your tongue up against the area in the back of the mouth where I showed you. 4. Please hold the back of your tongue up in that position for 3 seconds. 5. Please repeat this exercise 10 times.	1. Por favor abra su boca. 2. Voy a poner un depresor de lengua en su boca para enseñarle el área posterior de su lengua que debe tocar. 3. Por favor mueva lo de atrás de su lengua para arriba y contra el área de atrás de su lengua que le enseñe. 4. Por favor deténgalo atrás de su lengua para arriba por 3 segundos. 5. Por favor repita este ejercicio 10 veces.

Treatment for Oral Preparatory Phase Disorders Improving Range of Tongue Movement

Overview

Patients with oral preparatory phase dysphagia may not be able to adequately control the bolus in the oral cavity. This inability may be secondary to reduced range and coordination of tongue movements.

Protocols are provided for facilitation exercises and compensatory strategies that can help improve tongue movements necessary to hold the bolus in the oral cavity (Boshart, 1998; Ford, Grotz, Pomerantz, Bruno, & Flannery, 1974; Gangale, 1993; Lazarus, Logemann, Rademaker, Kahrilas, Pajak, Lazar, et al., 1993; Logemann, 1998; Murry & Carrau, 2006; Swigert, 2000):

Compensatory Swallow Therapy Exercises

- Circular Dry Gauze Chew Exercise
- Tongue Bowl Lift Exercise
- Tongue Bowl Slide Exercise

Rehabilitative Swallow Therapy Techniques

- Head Forward Position Strategy
- Food Hold Strategy

Treatment for Oral Preparatory Phase Disorders
Improving Range of Tongue Movement
Protocol 3.41 (English/Spanish)

Circular Dry Gauze Chew Exercise

The *Circular Dry Gauze Chew Exercise* is a set of procedures used to facilitate an adequate hold of the bolus in the oral cavity (Gangale, 1993; Logemann, 1998; Murry & Carrau, 2006).

General Procedures
- Prepare a 5-inch by 5-inch gauze.
- Moisten the gauze just slightly with water and then wring out the gauze.
- Place one end of the gauze inside the patient's mouth.
- Hold the other side of the gauze.
- Instruct the patient to move the gauze around in the mouth in a circular movement.
- Repeat this exercise 10 times.

Note to the Clinician
- As the patient progresses in therapy, the same exercise can be performed using the following items (Logemann, 1998):
  - A Lifesaver candy tied to a piece of thread
  - A Toothette swab that has been lightly dipped in cranberry or apple juice
- Finally, when gross manipulation of these two items has been achieved, have the patient chew a piece of gum (Ford, Grotz, Pomerantz, Bruno, & Flannery, 1974).
- It is important to ensure the patient is not at risk for aspiration before using these items in therapy.

Potential Benefits of This Exercise
- Increased tongue strength
- Increased tongue range
- Increased circular movement of the tongue to form the bolus
- Increased hold of the bolus

Protocols for Circular Dry Gauze Chew Exercise: *Explanation and Instruction to the Patient*		
	Explanation in English	**Explicación en Español**
Clinician	The Circular Dry Gauze Chew Exercise helps to increase circular movement of the tongue to form the bolus. This exercise may help you hold food in your mouth adequately.	Este Ejercicio de Gasa Seca y Circular le ayuda a aumentar el movimiento circular de su lengua para formar el bolo. Este ejercicio le puede ayudar a retener la comida en su boca adecuadamente.
	Instruction in English	**Instrucción en Español**
Clinician	1. I will put a piece of gauze in your mouth. 2. I will hold onto one side of the gauze strip. 3. Next, move the gauze strip around in your mouth in a clockwise fashion. 4. Please pretend that you are chewing a piece of food. 5. I will repeat this exercise 10 times.	1. Voy a ponerle un pedazo de gasa en su boca. 2. Voy a detener un lado del pedazo de la gasa. 3. Por favor mueva el pedazo de gasa alrededor en su boca en el sentido de las agujas del reloj. 4. Por favor pretenda que esta comiendo un pedazo de comida. 5. Por favor repita este ejercicio 10 veces.

Treatment for Oral Preparatory Phase Disorders
Improving Range of Tongue Movement
Protocol 3.42 (English/Spanish)

Tongue Bowl Lift Exercise

The *Tongue Bowl Lift Exercise* is a set of procedures used to facilitate an adequate hold of the bolus in the oral cavity (Boshart, 1998; Gangele, 1993; Logemann, 1998; Murry & Carrau, 2006; Swigert, 2000).

General Procedures
- Place the tip of the tongue depressor in the middle of the tongue.
- Instruct the patient to curl up the lateral margins of the tongue to form a "bowl."
- Repeat this exercise 10 times.

Potential Benefits of This Exercise
- Increased tongue strength
- Increased tongue range
- Increased hold of the bolus with the tongue

Protocols for Tongue Bowl Lift Exercise: *Explanation and Instruction to the Patient*		
	Explanation in English	**Explicación en Español**
Clinician	The Tongue Bowl Lift Exercise helps increase your tongue strength. This exercise helps you hold food adequately with your tongue.	Este Ejercicio de Formar un Tazón y Levantar la Lengua le ayuda a aumentar la fuerza de su lengua. Este ejercicio le ayuda a retener comida adecuadamente con su lengua.
	Instruction in English	**Instrucción en Español**
Clinician	1. I will place the tip of the tongue depressor in the middle of your tongue. 2. Please curl up the sides of your tongue so that it forms a bowl in the middle. 3. Please repeat this exercise 10 times.	1. Voy a poner la punta del depresor de lengua en medio de su lengua. 2. Por favor enrolle los lados de su lengua hacia arriba para que forme un tazón en medio. 3. Por favor repita este ejercicio 10 veces.

Treatment for Oral Preparatory Phase Disorders
Improving Range of Tongue Movement
Protocol 3.43 (English/Spanish)

Tongue Bowl Slide Exercise

The *Tongue Bowl Slide Exercise* is a set of procedures used to facilitate an adequate hold of the bolus in the oral cavity (Boshart, 1998).

General Procedures

- Instruct the patient to stick out the tongue.
- Apply pressure with a tongue depressor to the tip of the tongue.
- Slide the tongue depressor backward toward the middle of the patient's tongue; (this sliding action should cause the middle of the tongue to form a "bowl" as the sides of the tongue rise upward).
- Instruct the patient to hold this tongue position for 5 seconds.
- Repeat this exercise 10 times.

Potential Benefits of This Exercise

- Increased tongue strength
- Increased hold of the bolus with the tongue

Protocols for Tongue Bowl Slide Exercise: *Explanation and Instruction to the Patient*		
	Explanation in English	**Explicación en Español**
Clinician	The Tongue Bowl Slide Exercise helps increase your tongue strength. This exercise may help you to hold food appropriately with your tongue before you swallow.	Este Ejercicio de El Resbalado de La Lengua de Tazón le ayuda a aumentar la fuerza de su lengua. Este ejercicio le puede ayudar a retener comida apropiadamente con su lengua antes de que trague.
	Instruction in English	**Instrucción en Español**
Clinician	1. Please stick out your tongue. 2. I will place the tip of this tongue depressor onto the tip of your tongue. 3. Next, I will slide the tongue depressor back until I reach the middle of your tongue. 4. Your tongue should be in a bowl-like position. 5. Please hold this position for 5 seconds. 6. Please repeat this exercise on your tongue 10 times.	1. Por favor saque la lengua. 2. Voy a poner la punta del depresor de lengua sobre la punta de su lengua. 3. Luego, voy a resbalar el depresor hacia atrás hasta que llegue al medio de su lengua. 4. Debe de estar en una posición como un tazón. 5. Por favor detenga esta posición por 5 segundos. 6. Por favor repita este ejercicio 10 veces.

Treatment for Oral Preparatory Phase Disorders
Improving Range of Tongue Movement
Protocol 3.44 (English/Spanish)

Head Forward Position Strategy

The *Head Forward Position Strategy* is a set of procedures used to facilitate an adequate hold of the bolus in the oral cavity (Logemann, 1998).

General Procedures
- Instruct the patient to tilt the head forward slightly and downward (this will help keep the food in the anterior portion of the oral cavity).
- Have the patient lift the head to a neutral position in order to begin the swallow.
- Repeat this exercise throughout mealtimes.

Note to the Clinician
- Do not use this strategy with patients who cannot form an adequate lip seal or are not able to propel the bolus backward in the oral cavity.

Potential Benefits of This Strategy
- Increased management of the bolus
- Decreased oral residue
- Decreased amounts of food on the floor of the mouth

Protocols for Head Forward Position Strategy: *Explanation and Instruction to the Patient*		
	Explanation in English	**Explicación en Español**
Clinician	The Head Forward Position Strategy helps you keep the food in the front part of your mouth.	Esta Estrategia de Posición de la Cabeza Hacia Adelante le ayuda a retener la comida en el frente de su boca.
	Instruction in English	**Instrucción en Español**
Clinician	1. Please tilt your head forward slightly while you're eating. 2. Please lift your head to a neutral position and begin to swallow. 3. Please repeat this strategy every time you put food or liquid in your mouth.	1. Por favor incline su cabeza ligeramente hacia adelante mientras que coma. 2. Por favor levante su cabeza en la posición neutral y comience a tragar. 3. Por favor repita esta estrategia cada vez que se ponga comida o líquido en su boca.

Treatment for Oral Preparatory Phase Disorders
Improving Range of Tongue Movement
Protocol 3.45 (English/Spanish)

Food Hold Strategy

The *Food Hold Strategy* is a set of procedures used to facilitate an adequate hold of the bolus in the oral cavity (Lazarus, Logemann, Rademaker, Kahrilas, Pajak, Lazar, et al., 1993; Logemann, 1998).

General Procedures
- Instruct the patient to keep the food that is put in the mouth in the anterior part of the oral cavity.
- Have the patient hold the food or liquid against the anterior portion of the hard palate and the tongue.
- Repeat this strategy during mealtimes.

Note to the Clinician
- The food texture is key in this compensatory strategy because holding the food in the anterior part of the mouth does not allow it to be adequately chewed or moistened. So foods of a dry, solid consistency (e.g., crackers, hamburgers) are not appropriate—the food consistency must range from puree to soft diet (e.g., banana, soft breads).

Potential Benefits of This Strategy
- Increased management of the bolus
- Decreased oral residue
- Decreased amounts of food on the floor of the mouth

Protocols for Food Hold Strategy: *Explanation and Instruction to the Patient*		
	Explanation in English	**Explicaciones Español**
Clinician	The Food Hold Strategy helps you keep the food in the front part of your mouth.	Esta Estrategia de Sostener la Comida le ayuda a retener la comida en la parte de enfrente de su boca.
	Instruction in English	**Instrucción en Español**
Clinician	1. I will put a tongue depressor in your mouth and touch the area where I want you to keep your food. 2. Please take a bite of food and chew. 3. Please keep the food in the front of your mouth where I showed you. 4. Please begin to swallow. 5. Please repeat this strategy every time you put food into your mouth.	1. Voy a poner un depresor de lengua en su boca y voy a tocar el área donde quiero que retenga su comida. 2. Por favor tome un bocado de comida y mastique. 3. Por favor retenga la comida enfrente de su boca donde le enseñe. 4. Por favor comience a tragar. 5. Por favor repita esta estrategia cada vez que se ponga comida en su boca.

Section 4

Treatment for Oral Phase Dysphagia

Overview of the Oral Phase of Swallowing and Associated Disorders

The speech-language pathologist should determine which compensatory swallow therapy exercises and rehabilitative swallow therapy techniques to implement in the treatment of oral phase dysphagia. Considerations in planning the treatment program include the following factors: (a) components of the oral phase, (b) problems associated with the oral phase, (c) signs and symptoms of oral phase dysphagia, and (d) general treatment goals.

Components of the Oral Phase

The oral phase of the swallow consists of the following components:

- Closure of the lips for the labial seal
- Anterior to posterior movement of the tongue to propel the bolus posteriorly
- Movement in the cheeks to keep food out of the lateral sulcus
- Positioning of the sides and the tip of the tongue against the alveolar ridge
- Elevation of the soft palate so that the bolus can pass through the anterior faucial pillars
- Initiation of contact between the soft palate and the posterior pharyngeal wall to prevent food or liquid from coming out of the nasal cavity

Problems Associated with the Oral Phase

Potential problems related to the oral phase include:

- Apraxia of the mechanisms of swallowing
- Tongue thrust
- Reduced oral sensation
- Reduced tension of the lip and cheeks
- Reduced shaping of the tongue
- Reduced range of motion of the tongue
- Reduced tongue strength
- Reduced anterior to posterior tongue movement
- Reduced posterior tongue control
- Reduced anterior tongue control
- Reduced seal between the velum and the tongue
- Reduced tongue-palate contact

Signs and Symptoms of Dysphagia in the Oral Phase

Signs and symptoms associated with the oral phase of swallowing include:

- Premature loss of food or liquid into the pharynx
- Residue in the sulcus between the lips and the gums
- Residue in the sulcus between the gums and the cheeks
- Residue on the floor of the mouth
- Residue on the tongue
- Residue on the hard palate

General Treatment Goals for Patients with Oral Phase Dysphagia

General treatment goals related to the oral phase include the following:

- Increasing oral sensitivity
- Increasing anterior to posterior movement of the bolus
- Reducing premature loss of the bolus

Treatment for Oral Phase Dysphagia
Increasing Oral Sensitivity

Overview of the Oral Phase of Swallowing and Associated Disorders

Patients with oral phase dysphagia may exhibit reduced oral sensitivity. This deficit may be secondary to swallow apraxia. According to Logemann (1998), oral onset and oral transit of the swallow may be facilitated by using compensatory swallow therapy exercises to increase oral sensation.

This section outlines compensatory swallow therapy exercises that can be used to increase oral sensitivity in the oral cavity (Bove, Mansson, & Eliasson, 1998; Kaatzke-McDonald, App, Post, & Davis, 1996; Lazarus, Logemann, Rademaker, Kahrilas, Pajak, Lazar, et al., 1993; Logemann, 1998; Murry & Carrau, 2006; Logemann, Pauloski, Colangelo, Lazarus, Fujiu, & Kahrilas, 1995; Perlman, 1993; Rosenbek, Robins, Fishback, & Levine, 1991; Rosenbek, Robbins, Willford, Kirk, Schiltz, Sowell, et al., 1998; Sciortino, Liss, Case, Gerritsen, & Katz, 2003; Swigert, 2000).

Compensatory Swallow Therapy Exercises

The following compensatory swallow therapy exercises are described next:

* Large Bolus Strategy
* Textured Bolus Strategy
* Sour Bolus Strategy
* Cold Bolus Strategy
* Spoon Press Strategy
* Thermal-Stimulation Strategy

Treatment for Oral Phase Dysphagia
Increasing Oral Sensitivity
Protocol 4.1 (English/Spanish)

Large Bolus Strategy

The *Large Bolus Strategy* is a set of procedures used to increase oral sensitivity (Lazzarus, Logemann, Rademaker, Kahrilas, Pajak, Lazar, et al., 1993; Logemann, 1998).

General Procedures
- Present a bolus of larger volume to the patient (e.g., 1 full teaspoon).
- Use any one of the following food consistencies: applesauce, pudding, or thickened apple, cranberry, or orange juice.
- Repeat this strategy five times.

Note to the Clinician
- Use clinical judgement when deciding to implement this strategy into the patient's therapy program.
- Make sure that the patient is not at risk for aspiration when implementing this strategy into the treatment program.

Potential Benefits of This Strategy
- Increased sensory awareness of the tongue
- Increased onset of the swallow
- Increased trigger of the pharyngeal swallow

Protocol for Large Bolus Strategy: *Explanation and Instruction to the Patient*		
	Explanation in English	**Explicación en Español**
Clinician	This Large Bolus Strategy helps to increase the sensation in your tongue, to help you initiate your swallow.	Esta Estrategia de Bolo Grande le ayuda a aumentar la sensación en su lengua para ayudarle a iniciar su tragar.
	Instruction in English	**Instrucción en Español**
Clinician	1. I will place a teaspoon with more food on it inside of your mouth. 2. Please open your mouth and close your lips around the spoon. 3. Remove the food from the spoon. 4. Please swallow. 5. Please repeat this strategy five times.	1. Voy a ponerle una cuchara con más comida adentro de su boca. 2. Por favor abra su boca y cierre sus labios alrededor de la cuchara. 3. Quite la comida de la cuchara. 4. Por favor trague. 5. Por favor repita esta estrategia 5 veces.

Treatment for Oral Phase Dysphagia
Increasing Oral Sensitivity
Protocol 4.2 (English/Spanish)

Textured Bolus Strategy

The *Textured Bolus Strategy* is a set of procedures used to increase oral sensitivity (Lazzarus, Logemann, Rademaker, Kahrilas, Pajak, Lazar, et al., 1993; Logemann, 1998; Perlman, 1993; Swigert, 2000).

General Procedures
- Present a teaspoon of tapioca, pudding, or rice pudding to the patient.
- Repeat for five trials, or as many as the patient tolerates.

Note to the Clinician
- Use clinical judgement when deciding to implement this strategy into the patient's therapy program.
- The patient should be able to safely consume puree or pudding food consistencies before this compensatory strategy is implemented.

Potential Benefits of This Strategy
- Increased sensory awareness of the tongue
- Increased onset of the swallow

Protocol for Textured Bolus Strategy: *Explanation and Instruction to the Patient*		
	Explanation in English	**Explicación en Español**
Clinician	This Textured Bolus Strategy helps to increase the sensation in your tongue to help you initiate your swallow.	Esta Estrategia de Bolo con Textura le ayuda a aumentar la sensación en su lengua para ayudarle a iniciar su tragar.
	Instruction in English	**Instrucción en Español**
Clinician	1. I will put a teaspoon in your mouth with pudding/tapioca/rice pudding on it. 2. Please open your mouth so that I can put the spoon in your mouth. 3. Next, please close your lips around the spoon. 4. Remove the food from the spoon. 5. Please swallow now. 6. I will give you a teaspoon of pudding/tapioca/rice five times.	1. Voy a ponerle una cuchara en su boca con pudín /tapioca /atole de arroz. 2. Por favor abra la boca para que pueda ponerle la cuchara en su boca. 3. Por favor cierre sus labios alrededor de la cuchara. 4. Quite la comida de la cuchara. 5. Por favor trague. 6. Voy a darle una cucharada de pudín/ tapioca/atole de aroz cinco veces.

Treatment for Oral Phase Dysphagia
Increasing Oral Sensitivity
Protocol 4.3 (English/Spanish)

Sour Bolus Strategy

The *Sour Bolus Strategy* is a set of procedures used to increase oral sensitivity (Logemann, Pauloski, Colangelo, Lazarus, Fujiu, & Kahrilas, 1995; Swigert, 2000).

General Procedures
- Use regular or thickened acidic fruit juices such as lemon, lime orange, or grapefruit juice.
- Present a teaspoon containing a small amount of one of these juices.
- Repeat for five trials, or as many as the patient is able to tolerate.

Note to the Clinician
- Use clinical judgement when deciding to implement this strategy into the patient's program.
- The patient should be able to safely consume thickened juices before this strategy is implemented.

Potential Benefits of This Strategy
- Increased sensory awareness of the tongue
- Improved ability to initiate the swallow

Protocol for Sour Bolus Strategy: *Explanation and Instruction to the Patient*		
	Explanation in English	**Explicación en Español**
Clinician	This Sour Bolus Strategy helps to increase the sensation in your tongue, to help you initiate your swallow.	Esta Estrategia de Bolo Amargo le ayuda a aumentar la sensación en su lengua para ayudarle a iniciar el tragar.
	Instruction in English	**Instrucción en Español**
Clinician	1. I will put a teaspoon in your mouth with lemon/lime/orange/or grapefruit juice on it. 2. Please open your mouth so that I can put the spoon in your mouth. 3. Next, please close your lips around the spoon. 4. Remove the juice from the spoon. 5. Please swallow now. 6. I will give you a teaspoon of lemon/lime/orange/ or grapefruit juice for a total of five times. 7. Please swallow after every presentation of juice.	1. Voy a ponerle una cuchara en su boca con jugo de limón/lima/naranja/o toronja en ella. 2. Por favor abra su boca para que pueda poner la cuchara en su boca. 3. Por favor cierre sus labios alrededor de la cuchara. 4. Quite el jugo de la cuchara. 5. Por favor trague. 6. Le voy a dar una cucharada de jugo de limón/lima/naranja/o toronja por un total de cinco veces. 7. Por favor trague después de cada presentación de jugo.

Treatment for Oral Phase Dysphagia
Increasing Oral Sensitivity
Protocol 4.4 (English/Spanish)

Cold Bolus Strategy

The *Cold Bolus Strategy* is a set of procedures used to increase oral sensitivity (Logemann, 1998; Murry & Carrau, 2006).

General Procedures
- Present 1 teaspoon of applesauce or pudding that is cold.
- Repeat for as many trials as the patient tolerates without signs or symptoms of aspiration.

Note to the Clinician
- Do not use ice cream or frozen yogurt for the cold bolus. Ice cream and frozen yogurt melt once they get inside the mouth and turn into a thinner consistency.
- Use clinical judgement when deciding to include this strategy in the patient's therapy program.
- The patient should be able to safely ingest food of pureed consistency before implementation of this compensatory strategy.

Potential Benefits of This Strategy
- Increased sensory awareness of the tongue
- Increased the onset of the swallow
- Increased trigger of the pharyngeal swallow

Protocol for Cold Bolus Strategy: *Explanation and Instruction to the Patient*		
	Explanation in English	**Explicación en Español**
Clinician	The Cold Bolus Strategy helps to increase the sensation of your tongue, to help you initiate your swallow.	Esta Estrategia de Bolo Frió le ayuda a aumentar la sensación de su lengua para ayudarle a iniciar su tragar.
	Instruction in English	**Instrucción en Español**
Clinician	1. I will put a spoon with cold applesauce/pudding in your mouth. 2. The applesauce/pudding will be very cold. 3. I will give you a teaspoon with cold applesauce/pudding for a total of five times. 4. Please swallow after every presentation of applesauce/pudding.	1. Voy a ponerle una cuchara con puré de manzana /pudín frió en su boca. 2. El puré de manzana /pudín va a estar muy frió. 3. Voy a darle una cucharada con puré de manzana/pudín frió por un total de cinco veces. 4. Por favor trague después de cada presentación de puré de manzana/ pudín.

Treatment for Oral Phase Dysphagia
Increasing Oral Sensitivity
Protocol 4.5 (English/Spanish)

Spoon Press Strategy

The *Spoon Press Strategy* is a set of procedures used to increase oral sensitivity (Logemann, 1998; Swigert, 2000; Murry & Carrau, 2006)

General Procedures
- Place the teaspoon in the patient's mouth.
- Apply downward pressure against the patient's tongue.
- Continue this strategy with oral presentations of food to the patient.

Note to the Clinician
- Make sure that the patient is not at risk for aspiration before implementing this strategy.
- Use clinical judgement when deciding what type of food or liquid consistency to present to the patient.

Potential Benefits of This Strategy
- Increased sensory awareness of the tongue
- Increased initiation of the swallow

Protocol for Spoon Press Strategy: *Explanation and Instruction to the Patient*		
	Explanation in English	**Explicación en Español**
Clinician	The Spoon Press Strategy helps to increase sensation of your tongue so that you can initiate a swallow.	Esta Estrategia El Apretón de Cuchara le ayuda a aumentar la sensación de su lengua para que pueda iniciar un trago.
	Instruction in English	**Instrucción en Español**
Clinician	1. I will give you some food on a teaspoon. 2. Please open your mouth. 3. When I put the food in your mouth, I will apply pressure against your tongue with the spoon. 4. Please swallow. 5. Please use this strategy every time you take a bite of food.	1. Voy a darle comida en una cuchara. 2. Por favor abra la boca. 3. Cuando le ponga comida en su boca, voy a aplicarle presión contra su lengua con la cuchara. 4. Por favor trague. 5. Por favor use esta estrategia cada vez que tome un bocado de comida.

Treatment for Oral Phase Dysphagia
Increasing Oral Sensitivity
Protocol 4.6 (English/Spanish)

Thermal-Tactile Stimulation Exercise/Strategy

The *Thermal-Tactile Stimulation Exercise/Strategy* is a set of procedures used to increase oral sensitivity (Bove, Mansson, & Eliasson, 1998; Kaatzke-McDonald, App, Post, & Davis, 1996; Lazzara, Lazarus, & Logemann, 1986; Rosenbek, Robins, Fishback, & Levine, 1991; Rosenbek, Robbins, Willford, Kirk, Schiltz, Sowell, et al., 1998; Sciortino, Liss, Case, Gerritsen, & Katz, 2003).

General Procedures
- Use an iced lemon glycerine swab to perform the thermal-tactile stimulation.
- Instruct the patient to open the mouth.
- Place the iced lemon glycerin swab in the patient's mouth at the base of the anterior faucial pillars.
- Rub the right anterior faucial pillar up and down in a vertical movement.
- Ask the patient to swallow.
- Repeat this strategy five times on the right side.
- Repeat this procedure on the left side on the anterior faucial pillar five times.
- Present food to the patient (if used as a strategy) after thermal stimulation has been applied.
- Repeat this procedure three or four times a day for 5 to 10 minutes.

Potential Benefits of This Exercise/Strategy
- Improved initiation of the swallow reflex
- Increased stimulation in the oral cavity
- Increased sensory awareness

Protocol for Thermal-Tactile Stimulation Exercise/Strategy: *Explanation and Instruction to the Patient*

	Explanation in English	**Explicación en Español**
Clinician	This Thermal-Tactile Stimulation Exercise/Strategy helps to improve the initiation of your swallow. This exercise/strategy helps to increase the speed of your swallow.	Este Ejercicio/Estrategia de Estimulo Táctil le ayuda a mejorar la iniciación de su tragar. Este ejercicio/estrategia también le ayuda a aumentar la velocidad de su tragar.
	Instruction in English	**Instrucción en Español**
Clinician	1. I will place an iced swab in your mouth. 2. I will rub the iced swab on the right and left sides of the back of your throat. 3. Please open your mouth and keep it open. 4. I will place the iced swab on the right side of the back of your throat. 5. I will start at the bottom part of your throat and move upward. 6. I will repeat the same exercise/strategy on the left side. 7. I will complete this exercise/strategy five times on the both sides. 8. I will place food or liquid in your mouth (if used as a compensatory strategy). 9. Please swallow.	1. Voy a ponerle el aplicador de glicerina helado en su boca. 2. Voy a tallar el aplicador helado en el lado derecho y el lado izquierdo de atrás de su garganta. 3. Por favor abra su boca y mantengala abierta. 4. Voy a ponerle el aplicador helado en el lado derecho de atrás de su garganta. 5. Voy a comenzar en la parte de abajo de su garganta y moverme hacia arriba. 6. Voy a repetir este mismo ejercicio/estrategia en el lado izquierdo. 7. Voy a hacer este ejercicio/estrategia cinco veces en los dos lados. 8. Voy a ponerle comida o líquido en su boca. 9. Por favor trague.

Treatment for Oral Phase Dysphagia
Improving Anterior to Posterior Movement of the Bolus

Patients who exhibit oral phase dysphagia may have difficulty moving the bolus from the front of the oral cavity to the back of the oral cavity. This section outlines compensatory swallow therapy exercises and rehabilitative swallow therapy techniques that can be used with patients who exhibit decreased anterior to posterior movement of the bolus (Boshart, 1998; Buckley, Addicks, & Maniglia, 1976; Larsen, 1973; Lazarus, Logemann, Rademaker, Kahrilas, Pajak, Lazar, et al., 1993; Logemann, 1998; Murry & Carrau, 2006; Singh, Brockbank, Frost, & Tyler, 1995; Swigert, 2000).

Compensatory Swallow Therapy Exercises

The following compensatory swallow therapy exercises are described next:

- Tongue Squeeze Exercise
- Modified Tongue Squeeze Exercise
- Swab Swipe Exercise
- Tongue Tip Swipe Exercise
- Middle Tongue Pop Exercise

Rehabilitative Swallow Therapy Techniques

The following rehabilitative swallow therapy techniques also are described:

- Posterior Food Position Strategy
- Dump and Swallow Strategy
- Dump and Swallow with Supraglottic Swallow Strategy
- Food Hold Strategy
- Midline Food Position Strategy

Treatment for Oral Phase Dysphagia
Improving Anterior to Posterior Movement of the Bolus
Protocol 4.7 (English/Spanish)

Tongue Squeeze Exercise

The *Tongue Squeeze Exercise* is a set of procedures used to increase anterior to posterior movement of the bolus (Logemann, 1998).

General Procedures
- Prepare a piece of gauze that is 5 inches long.
- Place the tip of one side of the gauze into thickened apple, orange, or cranberry juice.
- Put one end of the gauze inside the patient's mouth while holding on to the other side of the gauze.
- Instruct the patient to push up and backward with the tongue and then move the piece of gauze upward against the roof of the mouth.
- Repeat this exercise five times.

Note to the Clinician
- Use clinical judgement when deciding to implement this exercise into the patient's therapy program.
- Make sure that the patient is not at risk for aspiration before implementing this exercise into the treatment program.

Potential Benefits of This Exercise
- Increased anterior to posterior movement of the bolus
- Increased tongue strength
- Increased tongue range

Protocol for Tongue Squeeze Exercise: *Explanation and Instruction to the Patient*		
	Explanation in English	**Explicación en Español**
Clinician	This Tongue Squeeze Exercise helps you move food and liquid from the front to the back of your mouth.	Este ejercicio de Apretón de Lengua le ayuda a mover la comida y líquido de la parte de enfrente a la parte de atrás de su boca.
	Instruction in English	**Instrucción en Español**
Clinician	1. I will place a piece of gauze in your mouth that has thickened cranberry/orange/apple juice. 2. I will hold the other side of the gauze. 3. Please close your lips. 4. Please move your tongue up and backward pressing the gauze against the roof of your mouth. 5. Please repeat this exercise five times.	1. Voy a ponerle un pedazo de gasa en su boca que tiene jugo espesado de arandano/naranja/manzana. 2. Voy a detener el otro lado de la gasa. 3. Por favor cierre sus labios. 4. Por favor mueva su lengua para arriba y para atrás empujando la gasa contra su paladar. 5. Por favor repita este ejercicio cinco veces.

Treatment for Oral Phase Dysphagia
Improving Anterior to Posterior Movement of the Bolus
Protocol 4.8 (English/Spanish)

Modified Tongue Squeeze Exercise

The *Modified Tongue Squeeze Exercise* is a set of procedures used to increase anterior to posterior movement of the bolus (Logemann, 1998).

General Procedures

- Prepare five 5-inch gauze strips and roll them up.
- Put the tip of the rolled gauze strips into thickened apple, orange, or cranberry juice.
- Place the end of the juice-moistened gauze strip into the patient's mouth.
- Hold on to the other end of the gauze strip.
- Instruct the patient to push upward against the gauze strip with the tongue and to move it backward.
- Have a tight grip on the other end of the gauze strip so that the patient does not swallow it.
- Adjust the amount of gauze strips as the patient's tongue elevation improves.
- Repeat this exercise five times.

Note to the Clinician

- Use clinical judgement when deciding to implement this exercise into the patient's therapy program.
- Make sure that the patient is not at risk for aspiration before implementing this exercise.
- The gauze strips can be made thinner as the patient's tongue elevation improves.

Potential Benefits of This Exercise

- Increased anterior to posterior movement of the bolus
- Increased tongue strength
- Increased tongue range

Protocol for Modified Tongue Squeeze Exercise: *Explanation and Instruction to the Patient*		
	Explanation in English	**Explicación en Español**
Clinician	This Modified Tongue Squeeze Exercise helps you move the food and liquid from the front to the back of your mouth.	Este Ejercicio de Apretón de Lengua Modificado le ayuda a mover la comida y líquido de la parte de enfrente a la parte de atrás de su boca.
	Instruction in English	**Instrucción en Español**
Clinician	1. I will place a thick piece of gauze in your mouth that has been dipped in thickened cranberry/orange/apple juice. 2. I will hold the other side of the gauze. 3. Please close your lips. 4. Please move your tongue up and backward, pressing the gauze against the roof of your mouth. 5. Please repeat this exercise five times.	1. Voy a ponerle un pedazo grueso de gasa en su boca que ha sido sumegido en jugo espesado de arandano/naranja/manzana. 2. Voy a detener el otro lado de la gasa. 3. Por favor cierre los labios. 4. Por favor mueva su lengua para arriba y para atrás empujando la gasa contra el paladar. 5. Por favor repita este ejercicio cinco veces.

Treatment for Oral Phase Dysphagia
Improving Anterior to Posterior Movement of the Bolus
Protocol 4.9 (English/Spanish)

Swab Swipe Exercise

The *Swab Swipe Exercise* is a set of procedures used to increase anterior to posterior movement of the bolus (Boshart, 1998).

General Procedures
- Place a lemon glycerin swab inside the patient's mouth on the tip of the tongue.
- Instruct the patient to move the tip of the glycerin swab up against the roof of the mouth with the tongue and move the swab backward with a rolling motion.
- Keep a tight grip on the handle of the swab, not allowing the patient to move it too far back with the tongue.
- Repeat this exercise five times.

Potential Benefits of This Exercise
- Increased anterior to posterior movement of the bolus
- Increased tongue strength and range

Protocol for Swab Swipe Exercise: *Explanation and Instruction to the Patient*		
	Explanation in English	**Explicación en Español**
Clinician	This Swab Swipe Exercise helps you move the food and liquid from the front to the back of your mouth.	Este Ejercicio de Limpiar con Aplicador le ayuda a mover la comida y líquido de la parte de enfrente a la parte de atrás de su boca.
	Instruction in English	**Instrucción en Español**
Clinician	1. I will place a swab in your mouth on the tip of your tongue. 2. I will hold the other side of the swab. 3. Please close your lips. 4. Please move your tongue up and back, pressing the swab against the roof of your mouth (in a rolling motion). 5. Please repeat this exercise five times.	1. Voy a poner un aplicador en su boca en la punta de su lengua. 2. Voy a detener el otro lado del aplicador. 3. Por favor cierre sus labios. 4. Por favor mueva su lengua para arriba y para atrás empujando contra el paladar (en un movimiento ondulante). 5. Por favor repita este ejercicio cinco veces.

Treatment for Oral Phase Dysphagia
Improving Anterior to Posterior Movement of the Bolus
Protocol 4.10 (English/Spanish)

Tongue Tip Swipe Exercise

The *Tongue Tip Swipe Exercise* is a set of procedures used to increase anterior to posterior movement of the bolus (Murry & Carrau, 2006; Swigert, 2000).

General Procedures

- Instruct the patient to put the tip of the tongue against the alveolar ridge and slide the tongue tip back against the hard palate and the soft palate.
- Repeat this exercise 10 times.

Potential Benefits of This Exercise

- Increased tongue tip strength
- Increased vertical movement of the tongue
- Increased tongue tip formation needed for initiation of swallowing
- Increased anterior to posterior movement of the tongue

Protocol for Tongue Tip Swipe Exercise: *Explanation and Instruction to the Patient*		
	Explanation in English	**Explicación en Español**
Clinician	This Tongue Tip Swipe Exercise will increase the strength in your tongue. This exercise may help you to hold the food in your mouth and move it back adequately before you swallow.	Este Ejercicio de Limpiar con la Punta de la Lengua le ayudará a aumentar la fuerza en su lengua. Este ejercicio le puede ayudar a retener la comida en su boca y moverla para atrás adecuadamente antes de que trague.
	Instruction in English	**Instrucción en Español**
Clinician	1. I will place a tongue depressor on the front part of the roof of your mouth [the clinician places the tongue depressor on the alveolar ridge]. 2. Please put the tip of your tongue on this spot. 3. Please slide your tongue backward along the roof of your mouth. Then relax and hold it in that position for 3 seconds. 4. Please slide your tongue tip forward along the roof of your mouth toward the front of your mouth. 5. Please repeat this exercise 10 times.	1. Voy a poner el depresor de lengua en frente del paladar de su boca [el clinico pone el depresor de lengua en el proceso alveolar]. 2. Por favor ponga la punta de su lengua en este punto. 3. Por favor resbale su lengua hacia atrás sobre el paladar y descanse y luego deténgala en esta posición por 3 segundos. 4. Por favor resbale la punta de su lengua hacia enfrente sobre el paladar hacia el frente de la boca. 5. Por favor repita este ejercicio 10 veces.

Treatment for Oral Phase Dysphagia
Improving Anterior to Posterior Movement of the Bolus
Protocol 4.11 (English/Spanish)

Middle Tongue Pop Exercise

The *Middle Tongue Pop Exercise* is a set of procedures used to increase anterior to posterior movement of the bolus (Boshart, 1998).

General Procedures
- Instruct the patient to slide the tip of the tongue toward the middle of the hard palate.
- Ask the patient to click the tip of the tongue against the middle portion of the palate.
- Complete 10 trials of this exercise.

Potential Benefits of This Exercise
- Increased tongue tip strength
- Increased tongue tip range
- Increased anterior to posterior movement of the tongue

Protocol for Middle Tongue Pop Exercise: *Explanation and Instruction to the Patient*		
	Explanation in English	**Explicación en Español**
Clinician	This Middle Tongue Pop Exercise helps you move your food back and forth in your mouth. This exercise may help you to move the food or liquid in your mouth more easily.	Este Ejercicio de Explosión con el Medio de la Lengua le ayuda a mover su comida para atrás y adelante en su boca. Este ejercicio le puede ayudar a mover la comida o líquido en su boca con más facilidad.
	Instruction in English	**Instrucción en Español**
Clinician	1. I will show you where I want you to click the tip of your tongue [the clinician shows the patient with a tongue depressor where to place the tip of the tongue on the hard palate]. 2. Please place your tongue behind your teeth and move it back toward the spot that I showed you. 3. Please click the tip of the tongue against the spot where I showed you. 4. Please repeat this exercise 10 times.	1. Voy a enseñarle donde quiero que haga clic con la punta de la lengua [el clinico le ensena al paciente con el depresor de lengua donde debe poner la punta de la lengua en el paladar]. 2. Por favor ponga su lengua atrás de sus dientes y muévala para atrás al punto que le enseñe. 3. Por favor haga clic con la punta de la lengua contra el punto que le enseñe. 4. Por favor repita este ejercicio 10 veces.

Treatment for Oral Phase Dysphagia
Improving Anterior to Posterior Movement of the Bolus
Protocol 4.12 (English/Spanish)

Posterior Food Position Strategy

The *Posterior Food Position Strategy* is a set of procedures used with patients who exhibit decreased anterior to posterior movement of the bolus (Logemann, 1998).

General Procedures
- Instruct the patient to place food on the posterior portion of the oral cavity.
- Complete this compensatory strategy during treatment sessions at the beginning.
- Implement this strategy at mealtimes.

Note to the Clinician
- Use clinical judgement when deciding to implement this strategy into the patient's therapy program.
- Make sure that the patient is not at risk for aspiration before implementing this strategy.
- Introduce this strategy when the patient is able to trigger the swallow reflex and exhibits appropriate mechanisms/behaviors for protection of the airway (Buckley, Addicks, & Maniglia, 1976).

Potential Benefits of This Strategy
- Increased control of the bolus
- Decreased residue in the oral cavity
- Decreased oral transit time

Protocol for Posterior Food Position Strategy: *Explanation and Instruction to the Patient*		
	Explanation in English	**Explicación en Español**
Clinician	This Posterior Food Position Strategy helps you move the food in the front of your mouth to the back of your mouth easier.	Esta Estrategia de Posición de la Comida en la Parte Posterior le ayuda a mover su comida para atrás y adelante en su boca. Esta estrategia le ayudará a mover la comida o líquido en su boca con más facilidad.
	Instruction in English	**Instrucción en Español**
Clinician	1. I will place your food on the back part of the tongue. 2. Please swallow. 3. Please use this strategy for every bite and at every meal.	1. Le voy a poner su comida en la parte de atrás de su lengua. 2. Por favor trague. 3. Por favor use esta estrategia para cada bocado y cada vez que coma.

Treatment for Oral Phase Dysphagia
Improving Anterior to Posterior Movement of the Bolus
Protocol 4.13 (English/Spanish)

Dump and Swallow Strategy

The *Dump and Swallow Strategy* is used by patients who exhibit decreased anterior to posterior movement of the bolus (Logemann, 1998; Singh, Brockbank, Frost, & Tyler, 1995; Swigert, 2000).

General Procedures
- Place food or liquid on the patient's tongue.
- Instruct the patient to tilt the head back to allow gravity to pull the food or liquid back.
- Implement this strategy into the patient's mealtimes if there are no signs or symptoms of aspiration.

Note to the Clinician
- Requirements for use of this strategy include the following (Logemann, 1998; Swigert, 2000):
  - ➢ The patient is cognitively coherent.
  - ➢ The patient is able to respond adequately to penetration in the airway (e.g., productive cough).
  - ➢ The patient is able to trigger the pharyngeal swallow appropriately.
  - ➢ The patient has adequate control of the larynx.
  - ➢ The patient does not exhibit pharyngeal phase dysphagia.

Potential Benefits of This Strategy
- Increased anterior to posterior movement of the bolus
- Decreased oral transit time
- Decreased need for tongue elevation if the patient is unable to achieve it (e.g., a patient with a glossectomy)

Protocol for Dump and Swallow Strategy: *Explanation and Instruction to the Patient*		
	Explanation in English	**Explicación en Español**
Clinician	This Dump and Swallow Strategy helps you move food from the front to the back of your mouth. This strategy may help you initiate a swallow.	Esta estrategia de Vertir y Tragar le ayuda a mover la comida de enfrente a lo de atrás de su boca. Esta estrategia le puede ayudar a iniciar el tragar.
	Instruction in English	**Instrucción en Español**
Clinician	1. Please put the food in your mouth. 2. Please tilt your head back. 3. Please swallow. 4. Please do this every time you put food in your mouth.	1. Por favor ponga la comida en su boca. 2. Por favor incline su cabeza hacia atrás. 3. Por favor trague. 4. Por favor haga esto cada vez que se ponga comida en la boca.

Treatment for Oral Phase Dysphagia
Improving Anterior to Posterior Movement of the Bolus
Protocol 4.14 (English/Spanish)

Dump and Swallow with the Supraglottic Swallow Strategy

The *Dump and Swallow* with the Supraglottic Swallow Strategy is a set of procedures used with patients who exhibit decreased anterior to posterior movement of the bolus (Larsen, 1973; Logemann, 1998).

General Procedures

- Instruct the patient to take a deep breath and to hold it.
- Give very small amounts of liquid (1 or 3 ml) on a spoon and instruct the patient to tilt the head backward while holding the breath.
- Instruct the patient to swallow 2–3 times or as many times as needed to clear the liquid while continuing to hold the breath.
- Instruct the patient to cough to clear any residue from the pharynx.

Note to the Clinician

- Implement this compensatory strategy only if there is adequate airway closure.
- Requirements for use of this strategy include the following (Logemann, 1998; Swigert, 2000):
  - ➢ The patient is cognitively coherent.
  - ➢ The patient is able to respond to penetration in the airway adequately (e.g., productive cough).
  - ➢ The patient is able to trigger the pharyngeal swallow appropriately.
  - ➢ The patient has adequate control of the larynx.

Potential Benefits of This Strategy

- Increased anterior to posterior movement of the bolus
- Decreased oral transit time
- Decreased need for tongue elevation if the patient is unable to achieve it (e.g., a patient with a glossectomy)

Protocol for Dump and Swallow with Supraglottic Swallow Strategy: *Explanation and Instruction to the Patient*		
	Explanation in English	**Explicación en Español**
Clinician	This Dump and Swallow Strategy with Supraglottic Swallow helps you move food from the front to the back of your mouth. This strategy may help you to initiate a swallow.	Esta Estrategia de Vertir y Tragar con un Supraglottic Trago le ayuda a mover la comida de enfrente a lo de atrás de su boca. Esta estrategia le puede ayudar a iniciar el tragar.
	Instruction in English	**Instrucción en Español**
Clinician	1. Please take a deep breath and hold it. 2. I will place small amounts of liquid in your mouth, please continue to hold your breath. 3. Please tilt your head back, while continuing to hold your breath. 4. Please swallow. 5. Please cough immediately after the swallow. 6. Please do this every time you put liquid in your mouth.	1. Por favor respire fuerte y deténgalo. 2. Voy a poner un poquito de liquido en su boca, continué deteniendo su respiración. 3. Por favor incline su cabeza hacia atrás mientras que detiene su respiración. 4. Por favor trague. 5. Por favor tosa inmediatamente después del trago. 6. Por favor haga esto cada vez que se ponga comida o líquido en su boca.

Treatment for Oral Phase Dysphagia
Improving Anterior to Posterior Movement of the Bolus
Protocol 4.15 (English/Spanish)

Food Hold Strategy

The *Food Hold Strategy* is a set of procedures used with patients who exhibit decreased anterior to posterior movement of the bolus (Lazarus, Logemann, Rademaker, Kahrilas, Pajak, Lazar, et al., 1993; Logemann, 1998).

General Procedures
- Instruct the patient to take a bite of food.
- Tell the patient to hold and push the food against the hard palate with the tongue.
- Instruct the patient to move the food with a single backward motion with the tongue and then swallow.
- Implement this strategy throughout meals if there are no signs or symptoms of aspiration.

Note to the Clinician
- Try this strategy during treatment sessions before instructing the patient to do this at every meal.
- Use clinical judgement when deciding to implement this strategy into the patient's therapy program.
- Ensure that the patient is not at risk for aspiration.
- This strategy most often is used with patients who have Parkinson's disease (Logemann, 1998).

Potential Benefits of This Strategy
- Increased tongue strength
- Increased tongue range
- Increased anterior to posterior movement of the bolus

Protocol for Food Hold Strategy: *Explanation and Instruction to the Patient*		
	Explanation in English	**Explicación en Español**
Clinician	This Food Hold Strategy helps you move food from the front to the back of your mouth.	Esta Estrategia de Sostener la Comida le ayuda a mover la comida de enfrente a la parte de atrás de su boca.
	Instruction in English	**Instrucción en Español**
Clinician	1. Please put some food in your mouth. 2. Please chew your food, moving it from one side of your mouth to the other side [if the patient has food that has texture]. 3. Please push the food upward with your tongue against the roof of your mouth. 4. Please move the food backward along the roof of your mouth with one backward slide of your tongue. 5. Please swallow. 6. Please complete this strategy five times. 7. Please use this strategy each time you put food into your mouth.	1. Por favor ponga comida en su boca. 2. Por favor mastique su comida moviendola de un lado de la boca al otro [si el paciente tiene comida con textura]. 3. Por favor empuje la comida hacia arriba con su lengua contra el paladar. 4. Por favor mueva la comida hacia atrás con un resbalo de la lengua sobre el paladar. 5. Por favor trague. 6. Por favor haga esta estrategia cinco veces. 7. Por favor use esta estrategia cada vez que se ponga comida en la boca.

Treatment for Oral Phase Dysphagia
Improving Anterior to Posterior Movement of the Bolus
Protocol 4.16 (English/Spanish)

Midline Food Position Strategy

The *Midline Food Position Strategy* is a set of procedures used with patients who exhibit decreased anterior to posterior movement of the bolus (Logemann, 1998; Swigert, 2000).

General Procedures
- Instruct the patient to place food on the middle portion of the tongue.
- Tell the patient to chew the food from side to side.
- Instruct the patient to move the food up and back against the hard palate with the tongue and swallow.
- Complete this compensatory strategy during treatment sessions.
- Implement this strategy at mealtimes.

Note to the Clinician
- Use this strategy with patients who can safely consume foods of puree or pudding consistency or finely chopped foods with sauce or gravy. These patients are able to keep the food on the midline of the tongue and then move it back into the oral cavity.
- Try this strategy during treatment sessions before instructing the patient to do this at every meal.
- Use clinical judgement when deciding to implement this strategy into the patient's therapy program.
- Make sure that the patient is not at risk for aspiration before implementing this strategy.

Potential Benefits of This Strategy
- Increased tongue strength
- Increased tongue range
- Increased anterior to posterior movement of the bolus
- Increased control of the bolus

Protocol for Midline Food Position Strategy: *Explanation and Instruction to the Patient*		
	Explanation in English	**Explicación en Español**
Clinician	This Midline Food Position Strategy helps you move the food from the front to the back of your mouth.	Esta estrategia de Posición de Comida en Medio de la Lengua le ayuda a mover la comida de enfrente a lo de atrás de su boca.
	Instruction in English	**Instrucción en Español**
Clinician	1. Please put some food in your mouth. 2. Please place the food on the middle of your tongue. 3. Please chew your food, moving it from one side of your mouth to the other side [if the patient has food that has texture]. 4. Please push the food upward with your tongue against the roof of your mouth. 5. Please move the food backward along the roof of your mouth. 6. Please swallow. 7. Please complete this strategy five times. 8. Please use this strategy each time you put food into your mouth.	1. Por favor ponga comida en su boca. 2. Por favor ponga la comida en medio de su lengua. 3. Por favor mastique su comida moviéndola de un lado de la boca al otro [si el paciente tiene comida con textura]. 4. Por favor empuje la comida hacia arriba contra el paladar. 5. Por favor mueva la comida hacia atrás sobre el paladar. 6. Por favor trague. 7. Por favor haga esta estrategia cinco veces. 8. Por favor haga esta estrategia cada vez que se ponga comida en la boca.

Treatment for Oral Phase Dysphagia
Improving Tongue Base Control

Overview

Many patients with oral phase dysphagia exhibit premature loss of the bolus secondary to weak control at the base of the tongue (Swigert, 2000). As a result, the patient is at risk for aspiration. The following section outlines compensatory swallow therapy exercises and rehabilitative swallow therapy techniques that can be used for patient who exhibit premature loss of the bolus (Bartolome & Neuman, 1993; Bryant, 1991; Bulow, Olsson, & Ekberg, 2001; Ding, Larson, Logemann, & Rademaker, 2002; Fujiu & Logemann, 1996; Gangale, 1993; Kahrilas, Logemann, Lin, & Ergun, 1992; Lazarus, Logemann, Song, Rademaker, & Kahrilas, 2002; Logemann, Kahrilas, Cheng, Pauloski, Gibbons, Rademaker, et al., 1992; Logemann, 1998; Murry & Carrau, 2006; Pounderoux & Kahrilas, 1995; Rasley, Logemann, Kahrilas, Rademaker, Pauloski, & Dodds, 1993; Shanahan, Logemann, Rademaker, Pauloski, & Kahrilas, 1993; Singh, Brockbank, Frost, & Tyler, 1995; Swigert, 2000; Welch, Logemann, Rademaker, & Kahrilas, 1993):

Compensatory Swallow Therapy Exercises

The following compensatory swallow therapy exercises are described next:

- Back Tongue Push-Up Exercise
- /k/ Tongue Productions Exercise
- Out/In Tongue Exercise
- Modified Tongue Tip Sweep Exercise
- Big Yawn Exercise
- Dry Gargle Exercise

Rehabilitative Swallow Therapy Techniques

The following compensatory strategies also are described:

- Tongue Anchor Exercise
- Mendelsohn Maneuver Exercise/Strategy
- Chin Tuck Strategy
- Reduced Bolus Size Strategy
- Effortful Swallow Exercise/Strategy
- Super-Supraglottic Swallow Exercise/Strategy

Treatment for Oral Phase Dysphagia
Improving Tongue Base Control
Protocol 4.17 (English/Spanish)

Back Tongue Push-up Exercise

The *Back Tongue Push-up Exercise* is used to improve tongue base control, to reduce the risk of premature spillage of the bolus into the pharynx (Swigert, 2000; Murry & Carrau, 2006).

General Procedures

- Show the patient with a tongue depressor the area of the soft palate where the back of the tongue should contact.
- Instruct the patient to push the back of the tongue up against the soft palate of the oral cavity.
- Have the patient place the tongue back in a /k/ position.
- Instruct the patient to hold this position for 3 seconds.
- Repeat this exercise 10 times.

Potential Benefits of This Exercise

- Increased strength of the back of the tongue
- Increased range of the back of the tongue
- Decreased premature spillage

Protocol for Back Tongue Push-up Exercise: *Explanation and Instruction to the Patient*		
	Explanation in English	**Explicación en Español**
Clinician	This Back Tongue Push-up Exercise helps to increase the strength in the back of your tongue. This exercise may prevent food or liquids from falling into your throat before you swallow.	Este Ejercicio de Levantar la Parte Posterior de la Lengua le ayuda a aumentar la fuerza de la parte posterior de la lengua. Este ejercicio puede evitar que la comida o líquidos se tiren en la garganta antes de que trague.
	Instruction in English	**Instrucción en Español**
Clinician	1. Please open your mouth. 2. I will place a tongue depressor in your mouth to show you what area the back of your tongue should touch. 3. Please move the back of your tongue up against the area in the back of the mouth where I showed you. 4. Please hold the back of your tongue up in that position for 3 seconds. 5. Please repeat this exercise 10 times.	1. Por favor abra su boca. 2. Voy a ponerle un depresor de lengua en su boca para enseñarle que área de su lengua debe tocar. 3. Por favor mueva la parte de atrás de su lengua para arriba contra el área de atrás de la lengua que le enseñe. 4. Por favor mantenga la parte de atrás de la lengua hacia arriba en esa posición por 3 segundos. 5. Por favor repita este ejercicio 10 veces.

Treatment for Oral Phase Dysphagia
Improving Tongue Base Control
Protocol 4.18 (English/Spanish)

/k/ Tongue Production Exercise

The */k/ Tongue Production Exercise* is a set of procedures used to increase strength in the back of the tongue, to reduce the risk of premature spillage of the bolus into the pharynx (Gangale, 1993; Murry & Carrau, 2006; Swigert, 2000).

General Procedures
- Instruct the patient to produce words with stress on the beginning phoneme /k/.
- Complete one list of words two times.

Note to the Clinician
- Check to see if the patient wears corrective lenses for vision before giving the patient the list.
- Say the word and then have the patient repeat the same word if the patient has visual or language impairments.

Potential Benefits of This Exercise
- Increased back of tongue control and strength
- Decreased premature spillage of the bolus

Protocol for /k/ Tongue Production Exercise: *Explanation and Instruction to the Patient*		
	Explanation in English	**Explicación en Español**
Clinician	This /k/ Tongue Production Exercise helps to increase the strength in the back of your tongue. This exercise may prevent food or liquids from falling into your throat before you swallow.	Este Ejercicio de Producción de Lengua con sonido /k/ le ayuda a aumentar la fuerza de atrás de la lengua. Este ejercicio puede evitar que la comida o líquidos se tiren en la garganta antes de que trague.
	Instruction in English	**Instrucción en Español**
Clinician	1. I will give you a list of words. 2. I will say some words to you. 3. Please repeat them aloud. 4. Please repeat the same words that I say. 5. When you say the words, please put emphasis on the beginning sound, which will be /k/. 6. Please repeat one list of words two times.	1. Voy a darle una lista de palabras. 2. Voy a decirle unas palabras a usted. 3. Por favor repitalas en voz alta. 4. Por favor repita las mismas palabras que yo dije. 5. Cuando diga las palabras ponga énfasis en el sonido primero, que será /k/. 6. Por favor repita una lista de palabras dos veces.

/k/ Word List in English

1. cab	16. cage	31. cop
2. calm	17. call	32. color
3. cane	18. came	33. college
4. car	19. can	34. cookie
5. case	20. cans	35. copy
6. coast	21. cape	36. court
7. cold	22. care	37. cub
8. cook	23. cart	38. kick
9. corn	24. cash	39. king
10. collar	25. camel	40. key
11. count	26. coat	41. kind
12. cut	27. cod	42. cough
13. kite	28. comb	43. cat
14. cup	29. cone	44. core
15. coal	30. cool	45. cow

/k/ Word List in Spanish

1. caqui	16. cantar	31. cambiar
2. cabra	17. cueva	32. cadera
3. caja	18. calle	33. caro
4. karate	19. carta	34. casa
5. coco	20. cachete	35. caer
6. cala	21. callo	36. caber
7. con	22. cama	37. camino
8. carro	23. caída	38. casar
9. cuento	24. cabello	39. caso
10. café	25. caballo	40. cabeza
11. costo	26. cada	41. causa
12. calcetín	27. cabaña	42. cara
13. kilo	28. camarón	43. cazo
14. calma	29. calar	44. coma
15. calcular	30. cargo	45. comer

Treatment for Oral Phase Dysphagia
Improving Tongue Base Control
Protocol 4.19 (English/Spanish)

Out/In Tongue Exercise

The *Out/In Tongue Exercise* is a set of procedures used to improve tongue base control, to reduce premature spillage of the bolus into the pharynx (Logemann, 1998; Murry & Carrau, 2006: Swigert, 2000).

General Procedures

- Instruct the patient to stick out the tongue as far as possible and then move the tongue backward as far as possible.
- Make sure the patient bunches up the tongue in the back of the throat (the patient should feel a sensation similar to gargling mouthwash or water).
- Repeat this exercise 10 times or for as many trials as the patient can tolerate.

Note to the Clinician

- Do not combine this exercise with protocols that present liquid or food.

Potential Benefits of This Exercise

- Increased tongue base range
- Increased tongue base strength
- Increased tongue base control

Protocol for Out/In Tongue Exercise: *Explanation and Instruction to the Patient*		
	Explanation in English	**Explicación en Español**
Clinician	This Out/In Tongue Exercise helps increase the strength in the back of your tongue. This exercise may prevent food or liquids from falling into your throat before you swallow.	Este Ejercicio de la Lengua para Fuera y Para Adentro le ayuda a aumentar la fuerza de atrás de la lengua. Este ejercicio puede evitar que la comida o líquidos desciendan en en su garganta antes de que trague.
	Instruction in English	**Instrucción en Español**
Clinician	1. Please stick out your tongue as far as possible. 2. Please move your tongue all the way to the back of your throat. 3. You will feel like your tongue is bunched up in the back of your throat, like when you gargle mouthwash or water. 4. Please repeat this exercise 10 times.	1. Por favor saque su lengua lo más que pueda. 2. Por favor mueva su lengua hacia atrás de su garganta completamente. 3. Sentirá que su lengua esta junta con la parte de atrás de la garganta como cuando se enjuaga uno la boca. 4. Por favor repita este ejercicio 10 veces.

Treatment for Oral Phase Dysphagia
Improving Tongue Base Control
Protocol 4.20 (English/Spanish)

Modified Tongue Tip Sweep Exercise

The *Modified Tongue Tip Sweep Exercise* is a set of procedures used to improve tongue base control, to decrease the risk of premature spillage of the bolus into the pharynx (Murry & Carrau, 2006).

General Procedures
- Instruct the patient to put the tip of the tongue against the alveolar ridge and then slide the tongue tip back against the hard palate and the soft palate.
- Tell the patient to stiffen the tongue in the back of the mouth as much as possible and hold that position for 2 seconds.
- Repeat this exercise 10 times.

Potential Benefits of This Exercise
- Increased tongue base control
- Increased tongue base strength

Protocol for Modified Tongue Tip Sweep Exercise: *Explanation and Instruction to the Patient*		
	Explanation in English	**Explicación en Español**
Clinician	This Modified Tongue Tip Sweep Exercise helps to increase the strength in the back of your tongue. This exercise may prevent food or liquids from falling into your throat before you swallow.	Este Ejercicio le ayuda a aumentar la fuerza de atrás de la Lengua. Este ejercicio puede evitar que la comida o líquidos desciendan en su garganta antes de que trague.
	Instruction in English	**Instrucción en Español**
Clinician	1. I will place a tongue depressor on the front of the roof of your mouth [the clinician places the tongue depressor on the alveolar ridge]. 2. Please put the tip of your tongue on this spot. 3. Please slide your tongue backward along the roof of your mouth then hold it in that position for 2 seconds, making your tongue as stiff as you can. 4. Please relax your tongue. 5. You will feel the muscles in the back of your throat moving. 6. Please repeat this exercise 10 times.	1. Voy a poner un depresor de lengua enfrente de su paladar [el clinico pone el depresor de lengua en el proceso alveolar]. 2. Por favor ponga la punta de su lengua en ese punto. 3. Por favor resbale su lengua hacia atrás sobre el paladar y deténgala en esa posición por 2 segundos, haciendo que su lengua se ponga tan dura como pueda. 4. Por favor descanse su lengua. 5. Sentirá los músculos de atrás de su garganta moviendose. 6. Por favor repita este ejercicio 10 veces.

Treatment for Oral Phase Dysphagia
Improving Tongue Base Control
Protocol 4.21 (English/Spanish)

Big Yawn Exercise

The *Big Yawn Exercise* is used to improve tongue base control, to decrease the risk of premature spillage of the bolus into the pharynx (Logemann, 1998; Swigert, 2000).

General Procedures
- Instruct the patient to yawn as wide as possible (this maneuver will facilitate the upward movement of the base of the tongue).
- Ask the patient to hold the yawn for 2 seconds.
- Repeat this exercise five times.

Potential Benefits of This Exercise
- Increased tongue base control
- Increased tongue base strength

Protocol for Big Yawn Exercise: *Explanation and Instruction to the Patient*		
	Explanation in English	**Explicación en Español**
Clinician	This Big Yawn Exercise helps to increase the strength in the back of your tongue. This exercise may prevent food or liquids from falling into your throat before you swallow.	Este Ejercicio de Bostezo Grande le ayuda a aumentar la fuerza de atrás de la Lengua. Este ejercicio puede evitar que la comida o líquidos desciendan en su garganta antes de que trague.
	Instruction in English	**Instrucción en Español**
Clinician	1. Please yawn as wide as possible. 2. Please keep yawning for 2 seconds. 3. Please repeat this exercise five times.	1. Por favor bosteze lo más ancho que pueda. 2. Por favor siga bostezeando por 2 segundos. 3. Por favor repita este ejercicio cinco veces.

Treatment for Oral Phase Dysphagia
Improving Tongue Base Control
Protocol 4.22 (English/Spanish)

Dry Gargle Exercise

The *Dry Gargle Exercise* is a set of procedures used to improve tongue base control, to decrease the risk of premature spillage of the bolus into the pharynx (Logemann, 1998: Swigert, 2000).

General Procedures
* Instruct the patient to pretend to gargle.
* Have the patient pretend to gargle for 5 seconds.
* Repeat this exercise 10 times.

Note to the Clinician
* Do not present any water or mouthwash to the patient for this exercise.

Potential Benefits of This Exercise
* Increased tongue base control
* Increased tongue base strength

Protocol for Dry Gargle Exercise: *Explanation and Instruction to the Patient*		
	Explanation in English	**Explicación en Español**
Clinician	This Dry Gargle Exercise helps to increase the strength in the back of your tongue. This exercise may prevent food or liquids from falling into your throat before you swallow.	Este Ejercicio de Gárgara Seca le ayuda a aumentar la fuerza de atrás de la Lengua. Este ejercicio puede evitar que la comida o líquidos desciendan en su garganta antes de que trague.
	Instruction in English	**Instrucción en Español**
Clinician	1. Please pretend that you are gargling with mouthwash or water. 2. Please gargle for 5 seconds. 3. Please repeat this exercise 10 times.	1. Por favor pretenda que esta gargareando con enjuague o agua. 2. Por favor gargaricé por 5 segundos. 3. Por favor repita este ejercicio 10 veces.

Treatment for Oral Phase Dysphagia
Improving Tongue Base Control
Protocol 4.23 (English/Spanish)

Tongue Anchor Exercise/Masako Maneuver

The *Tongue Anchor Exercise*, also known as the Masako maneuver, is a set of procedures used to improve tongue base control, to reduce the risk of premature spillage of the bolus into the pharynx (Fujiu & Logemann, 1996; Lazarus, Logemann, Song, Rademaker, & Kahrilas, 2002; Murry & Carrau, 2006; Swigert, 2000).

General Procedures
- Instruct the patient to stick out the tongue.
- Have the patient gently hold onto the tongue with the teeth.
- Tell the patient to swallow while holding onto the tongue with the teeth.
- Repeat this exercise 10 times.

Potential Benefits of This Exercise
- Increased tongue base control
- Increased tongue base strength

Protocol for Tongue Anchor Exercise: *Explanation and Instruction to the Patient*		
	Explanation in English	**Explicación en Español**
Clinician	This Tongue Anchor Exercise helps to increase the strength in the back of your tongue. This exercise may prevent food or liquids from falling into your throat before you swallow.	Este Ejercicio Modificado de Anclar la Lengua le ayuda a aumentar la fuerza de atrás de la lengua. Este ejercicio puede evitar que la comida o líquidos desciendan en su garganta antes de que trague.
	Instruction in English	**Instrucción en Español**
Clinician	1. Please stick the front part of your tongue outside of the mouth. 2. Please gently bite down on your tongue. 3. Please continue holding your tongue and swallow. 4. Please repeat this exercise 10 times.	1. Por favor saque la parte de enfrente de su lengua. 2. Por favor muerda su lengua suavemente. 3. Por favor continué deteniendo su lengua y trague. 4. Por favor repita este ejercicio 10 veces.

Treatment for Oral Phase Dysphagia
Improving Tongue Base Control
Protocol 4.24 (English/Spanish)

Mendelsohn Maneuver Exercise/Strategy

The *Mendelsohn Maneuver Exercise/Strategy* is a set of procedures used to increase extent and duration of laryngeal elevation. When the larynx is most elevated, the tongue base is also elevated and stays in contact with the pharyngeal wall; this action helps control the tongue base to decrease the risk of premature spillage of the bolus into the pharynx (Bartolome & Neuman, 1993; Bryant, 1991; Ding, Larson, Logemann, & Rademaker, 2002; Logemann, Kahrilas, Cheng, Pauloski, Gibbons, Rademaker, et al., 1992; Lazarus, Logemann, Song, Rademaker, & Kahrilas, 2002).

General Procedures
- Instruct the patient where to put the hand on the larynx (do not have the patient squeeze the larynx).
- Tell the patient to swallow [if using the Mendelsohn maneuver as a strategy, the clinician presents food or liquids].
- Show the patient when the larynx elevates.
- Instruct the patient to swallow and then have the patient identify the highest point when the larynx is elevated.
- Repeat this exercise five times.
- Instruct the patient to put the hand on the larynx and swallow.
- Have the patient identify the highest point of the larynx during the swallow and squeeze the muscles in the back of the tongue as hard and as long as possible without allowing the larynx to come back down.
- Repeat this exercise 10 times.

Note to the Clinician
- This initially is done as an exercise/strategy and then is implemented as a rehabilitative swallow maneuver while the patient is eating.

Potential Benefits of This Exercise
- Decreases pooling at the level of the pyriform sinuses
- Maintains opening of the cricopharyngeus for a longer period of time
- Increases coordination of the whole swallowing sequence
- Enhances the opening of the upper esophageal sphincter

Protocol for Mendelsohn Maneuver Exercise/Strategy: *Explanation and Instruction to the Patient*

	Explanation in English	Explicación en Español
Clinician	This Mendelsohn Maneuver Exercise/Strategy helps to increase the strength in the back of your tongue. This exercise/strategy may prevent food or liquids from falling into your throat before you swallow.	Este Ejercicio/Estrategia de Maniobra de Mendelsohn le ayuda a aumentar la fuerza de atras de la lengua. Este ejercicio/estrategia puede evitar que la comida o líquidos desciendan en su garganta antes de que trague.
	Instruction in English	**Instrucción en Español**
Clinician	1. Please put your hand on your throat. 2. I will put some food in your mouth [if the Mendelsohn Maneuver is being used as a compensatory strategy]. 3. Please swallow and feel your larynx go up. 4. Now, please show me with your hand where the larynx goes up the highest. 5. Now, please swallow. When your larynx reaches the highest point, please squeeze the back muscles of your tongue for as long and as hard as you can without letting your larynx go down. 6. Please repeat this exercise/strategy five times.	1. Por favor ponga su mano en su garganta. 2. Voy a poner comida en su boca. 3. Por favor trague y sienta su laringe cuando se mueve para arriba. 4. Luego, quiero que me enseñe con su mano donde la laringe se alzo lo más alto. 5. Por favor trague, Cuando su laringe llegue al punto más alto, quiero que apriete los músculos de atras de su lengua lo más largo y fuerte que pueda sin dcjar ir la laringe para abajo. 6. Por favor repita este ejercicio/estrategia cinco veces.

Treatment for Oral Phase Dysphagia
Improving Tongue Base Control
Protocol 4.25 (English/Spanish)

Chin Tuck Strategy

The *Chin Tuck Strategy* is a set of procedures used to improve tongue base control, to decrease the risk of premature spillage of the bolus (Bulow, Olsson, & Ekberg, 2001; Rasley, Logemann, Kahrilas, Rademaker, Pauloski, & Dodds, 1993; Shanahan, Logemann, Rademaker, Pauloski, & Kahrilas, 1993; Singh, Brockbank, Frost, & Tyler, 1995; Swigert, 2000; Welch, Logemann, Rademaker, & Kahrilas, 1993).

General Procedures
- Instruct the patient to move the head down and move the chin down toward the chest every time food or liquid is swallowed.
- Implement this strategy every time the patient consumes food or liquid.

Note to the Clinician
- Make sure that the patient is sitting up at a 90-degree angle.
- Also make sure that the patient is tucking the chin down and not leaning the head forward (Swigert, 2000).

Potential Benefits of This Strategy
- Increased back of tongue control
- Increased control of the bolus
- Decreased premature spillage into the pharynx

Protocol for Chin Tuck Strategy: *Explanation and Instruction to the Patient*		
	Explanation in English	**Explicación en Español**
Clinician	This Chin Tuck Strategy helps with control to the back of your tongue. This strategy may prevent food or liquids from falling into your throat before you swallow.	Esta Estrategia de Barbilla Hacia Abajo le ayuda a controlar la fuerza de atrás de la lengua. Esta estrategia puede evitar que la comida o líquidos desciendan en su garganta antes de que trague.
	Instruction in English	**Instrucción en Español**
Clinician	1. Please sit up as straight as possible. 2. Please put some food in your mouth. 3. Please move your head and chin down toward your chest. 4. Please swallow. 5. Please complete this strategy every time you swallow.	1. Por favor siéntese lo más derecho que pueda. 2. Por favor ponga comida en su boca. 3. Por favor mueva su cabeza y barbilla hacia su pecho. 4. Por favor trague. 5. Por favor haga esta estrategia cada vez que traga.

Treatment for Oral Phase Dysphagia
Improving Tongue Base Control
Protocol 4.26 (English/Spanish)

Reduced Bolus Size Strategy

The *Reduced Bolus Size Strategy* is a set of procedures used with patients who exhibit premature spillage of the bolus (Lazarus, Logemann, Rademaker, Kahrilas, Pajak, Lazar, et al., 1993; Swigert, 2000).

General Procedures
- Instruct the patient or caregiver to use a teaspoon or pediatric spoon for ingesting food and liquids (this may help control the amount of food or liquid that goes into the mouth).
- Tell the patient or caregiver how much food or liquid should be placed on the teaspoon (this amount will vary from patient to patient).
- Use clinical judgement when deciding how much food or liquid should go on the teaspoon or pediatric spoon.
- The patient uses this strategy during mealtimes.

Note to the Clinician
- Use clinical judgement when deciding to implement this strategy into the patient's therapy program.
- Make sure that the patient is not at risk for aspiration before implementing this strategy.

Potential Benefits of This Strategy
- Increased control of the bolus
- Decreased amount of bolus that goes into the oral cavity
- Decreased premature spillage of the bolus into the pharynx

Protocol for Reduced Bolus Size Strategy: *Explanation and Instruction to the Patient*		
	Explanation in English	**Explicación en Español**
Clinician	This Reduced Bolus Size Strategy helps to prevent food or liquids from falling into your throat before you swallow.	Esta Estrategia de Bolo Reducido en Tamaño le ayuda a evitar que la comida o líquidos entren a su garganta antes de que trague.
	Instruction in English	**Instrucción en Español**
Clinician	1. Please use a teaspoon or small spoon to eat with. 2. I will show you how much food or liquid I want you to put on your spoon every time you swallow. 3. This is the kind of spoon I want you to use and this is the amount of food and liquid I want you to put on the spoon every time you put food or liquid in your mouth. 4. Please use this strategy for every meal.	1. Por favor use una cuchara para comer. 2. Le voy a enseñar que tanta comida o líquido quiero que se ponga en la cuchara coda vez que trague. 3. Esta es la clase de cuchara que quiero que use y esta es la cantidad de comida o líquido que quiero que ponga en la cuchara cada vez que se ponga comida o líquido en su boca. 4. Quiero que use esta estrategia a cada vez que coma.

Treatment for Oral Phase Dysphagia
Improving Tongue Base Control
Protocol 4.27 (English/Spanish)

Effortful Swallow Exercise/Strategy

The *Effortful Swallow Exercise/Strategy* is a set of procedures used to improve tongue base control, to decrease the risk of premature spillage of the bolus into the pharynx (Kahrilas, Logemann, & Gibbons, 1992; Kahrilas, Logemann, Lin, & Ergun, 1992; Swigert, 2000; Pounderoux & Kahrilas, 1995).

General Procedures
- Instruct the patient to put some food or liquid inside the mouth.
- Tell the patient to squeeze and push the tongue backward as much as possible while swallowing (Swigert, 2000).
- The patient uses this strategy during mealtimes.

Note to the Clinician
- Use clinical judgement when deciding to implement this exercise/strategy into the patient's therapy program.
- Make sure that the patient is not at risk for aspiration before implementing this strategy.

Potential Benefits of This Exercise/Strategy
- Increased tongue base control
- Decreased premature spillage of the bolus into the pharynx

Protocol for Effortful Swallow Exercise/Strategy: *Explanation and Instruction to the Patient*		
	Explanation in English	**Explicación en Español**
Clinician	This Effortful Swallow Exercise/Strategy helps to prevent food or liquids from falling into your throat before you swallow.	Este Ejercicio/Estrategia de Trago con Esfuerzo le ayuda a evitar que la comida o los líquidos entren a su garganta antes de que trague.
	Instruction in English	**Instrucción en Español**
Clinician	1. Please place some food or liquid into your mouth. 2. Please chew your food [if the patient's food requires chewing] . 3. Please push and squeeze your tongue backward as hard as you can while you swallow. 4. Please complete this exercise/strategy every time you swallow.	1. Por favor ponga comida o líquido en su boca. 2. Por favor mastique su comida [si la comida del paciente requiere ser masticada]. 3. Por favor empuje y aplane su lengua hacia atrás lo más fuerte que pueda mientras que traga. 4. Por favor haga esteejercicio/estrategia cada vez que trague.

Treatment for Oral Phase Dysphagia
Improving Tongue Base Control
Protocol 4.28 (English/Spanish)

Super-Supraglottic Swallow Exercise/Strategy

The *Super-Supraglottic Swallow Exercise/Strategy* is a set of procedures used to improve tongue base control, to decrease the risk of spillage of the bolus into the pharynx (Donzelli & Brady, 2004; Kahrilas, Logemann, & Gibbons, 1992; Logemann, Pauloski, Rademaker, & Colangelo, 1997b; Martin, Logemann, Shaker, & Dodds, 1993; Swigert, 2000).

General Procedures
- Implement this exercise/strategy to increase tongue base control in patients who have had a supraglottic laryngectomy (Logemann, 1998).
- Have the patient do this exercise/strategy without presentation of food.
- Introduce food while incorporating this exercise/strategy.
- Instruct the patient to take a deep breath in and then exhale a little bit of air out.
- Tell the patient to hold the breath in as tightly as possible.
- Place food or liquid into the oral cavity (the patient should still be holding in the breath).
- Instruct the patient to continue holding the breath while squeezing as hard as possible during the swallow.
- Tell the patient to cough and then swallow again (Swigert, 2000).

Note to the Clinician
- Use clinical judgement when deciding to implement this exercise/strategy into the patient's therapy program.
- Make sure that the patient is not at risk for aspiration before implementing this exercise/ strategy.

Potential Benefits of This Exercise/Strategy
- Increased laryngeal closure in case premature spillage occurs
- Increased tongue base control

Protocol for Super-Supraglottic Swallow Strategy: *Explanation and Instruction to the Patient*		
	Explanation in English	**Explicación en Español**
Clinician	This Super-Supraglottic Swallow Exercise/Strategy helps prevent food or liquids from falling into your throat before you swallow.	Este Ejercicio/Estrategia de Trago Súper-Supraglottic le ayuda a evitar que la comida o líquidos entren a su garganta antes de que trague.
	Instruction in English	**Instrucción en Español**
Clinician	1. Please take a deep breath in and then exhale a little bit of air out. 2. Please hold the rest of the air in and don't let go of it. 3. I will put some food in your mouth. 4. Please continue holding your breath and squeeze while you are swallowing your food. 5. Please cough [once the patient finishes swallowing the food]. 6. Please swallow again.	1. Por favor respire y luego deje salir un poco de aire para afuera. 2. Por favor detenga el resto del aire y no lo deje salir. 3. Voy a poner comida en su boca. 4. Por favor continué deteniendo su respiración y apriete hacia abajo mientras que traga su comida. 5. Por favor tosa [después de que el paciente termine de tragar la comida]. 6. Por favor trague otra vez.

Section 5

Treatment for Pharyngeal and Esophageal Phases of Dysphagia

Overview of the Pharyngeal Phase of Swallowing and Associated Disorders

The speech-language pathologist should determine which compensatory swallow therapy exercises and rehabilitative swallow therapy strategies to implement in the treatment of pharyngeal phase dysphagia. Considerations in planning the treatment program include the following factors: (a) components of the pharyngeal phase, (b) problems associated with the pharyngeal phase, (c) signs and symptoms of pharyngeal phase dysphagia, and (d) general treatment goals.

Components of the Pharyngeal Phase

The pharyngeal phase of the swallow consists of the following components, as summarized from the work of Groher (1992), Logemann (1993, 1998), and Leonard and Kendall (1997):

- The tip of the bolus passes anywhere between the anterior faucial pillars and the point where the tongue base crosses the lower edge of the mandible.
- The velum elevates and moves back to close of the nasopharynx so that food or liquid does not come out of the nose.
- The larynx and hyoid bone elevate.
- The closure of the larynx occurs at the level of the true vocal folds, false vocal folds, and the epiglottis.
- The cricopharyngeal sphincter opens, allowing food and liquid to move from the pharynx to the esophagus.
- The base of the tongue moves up and back.
- The base of the tongue moves toward the posterior pharyngeal wall to deliver food or liquid to the pharynx.
- The tongue base retracts to contact the posterior pharyngeal wall.
- The pharyngeal sphincters contract from the top to the bottom.

Problems Associated with the Pharyngeal Phase

Potential problems related to the pharyngeal phase include the following:

- Delayed initiation of the pharyngeal swallow
- Decreased pharyngeal contraction
- Decreased vocal fold adduction
- Decreased tongue base movement
- Decreased posterior pharyngeal wall movement
- Decreased laryngeal elevation
- Decreased laryngeal closure

Signs and Symptoms That May Occur in the Pharyngeal Phase

Signs and symptoms of pharyngeal phase dysphagia include the following:

- Nasal regurgitation
- Coughing during the swallow
- Coughing after the swallow
- Clearing the throat during the swallow
- Clearing the throat after the swallow
- Increased wetness in the patient's voice after the swallow
- Increased congestion
- Difficulty taking medications because they get stuck in the throat
- Increased residue in the pharynx
- Increased residue in the valleculae
- Penetration of food or liquid into the airway
- Aspiration of food or liquid into the airway
- Increased residue in the pyriform sinuses

General Treatment Goals for Patients with Oral Phase Dysphagia

General treatment goals related to the pharyngeal phase include the following:

- Increasing the trigger of the pharyngeal phase of the swallow
- Reducing residue in the valleculae
- Reducing residue in the pharynx
- Increasing laryngeal closure of the airway
- Increasing laryngeal elevation

Treatment for Pharyngeal Phase Dysphagia
Improving Initiation of the Pharyngeal Swallow

Overview

Patients with pharyngeal phase dysphagia may have difficulty initiating the swallow reflex. As a result, the main portion of the bolus passes into the pharynx without the initiation of the swallow. Delay in the initiation of the swallow is different than premature entry of the bolus seen in the oral phase of the swallow. Premature spillage is when a small part of the bolus spills over the base of the tongue. The following section outlines rehabilitative swallow therapy strategy and compensatory swallow therapy strategies/exercises that can be used with patients who exhibit delayed initiation of the swallow reflex (Logemann, 1998; Murry & Carrau, 2006):

Rehabilitative Swallow Therapy Strategy

The following rehabilitative swallow therapy exercise/strategy is described next:

- Chin Down Strategy

Compensatory Swallow Therapy Strategies/Exercises

The following compensatory swallow therapy strategies/exercises also are described:

- Thermal-Tactile Stimulation Exercise/Strategy
- Suck Swallow Exercise
- Textured Bolus Strategy
- Sour Bolus Strategy
- Cold Bolus Strategy
- Small Bolus Strategy

Treatment for Pharyngeal Phase Dysphagia
Improving Initiation of the Pharyngeal Swallow
Protocol 5.1 (English/Spanish)

Chin Down Strategy

The *Chin Down Strategy* is a procedure used with patients who exhibit a delayed or absent trigger of the pharyngeal swallow reflex (Bulow, Olsson, & Ekberg, 2001; Rasley, Logemann, Kahrilas, Rademaker, Pauloski, & Dodds, 1993; Welch, Logemann, Rademaker, & Kahrilas, 1993).

General Procedures
- Instruct the patient to move the head down and move the chin down toward the chest when swallowing.
- Implement this strategy every time the patient consumes food or liquid.

Note to the Clinician
- Make sure that the patient is sitting up at a 90-degree angle.
- Also make sure that the patient is tucking the chin down and not leaning the head forward (Swigert, 2000).

Potential Benefits of This Strategy
- Increased back of tongue control
- Increased control of the bolus
- Reduced risk for aspiration and choking

Protocol for Chin Down Strategy: *Explanation and Instruction to the Patient*		
	Explanation in English	**Explicación en Español**
Clinician	This Chin Down Strategy helps to increase the strength in the back of your tongue and throat. This strategy may prevent food or liquids from falling into your throat or airway.	Esta Estrategia de Barbilla Hacia Abajo le ayuda a aumentar la fuerza en lo de atras de su lengua y su garganta. Esta estrategia le puede ayudar a evitar que entre comida o líquido a la garganta o la vía respiratoria.
	Instruction in English	**Instrucción en Español**
Clinician	1. Please sit up as straight as possible. 2. Please put some food in your mouth. 3. Please move your head and chin down toward your chest and swallow. 4. Please complete this strategy every time you put food or liquid into your mouth.	1. Por favor siéntese derecho todo lo que sea posible. 2. Por favor ponga la comida en su boca. 3. Por favor mueva su cabeza y su barbilla hacia abajo a su pecho y trague. 4. Por favor use esta estrategia cada vez que se ponga comida o líquido en su boca.

Treatment for Pharyngeal Phase Dysphagia
Improving Initiation of the Pharyngeal Swallow
Protocol 5.2 (English/Spanish)

Thermal-Tactile Stimulation Exercise/Strategy

The *Thermal-Tactile Stimulation Exercise/Strategy* is a set of procedures used with patients who exhibit delayed or absent triggering of the pharyngeal swallow (Bove, Marisson, & Eliasson, 1998; Rosenbek, Robbins, Willford, Kirk, Schiltz, Sowell, et al., 1998; Sciortino, Liss, Case, Gerritsen, & Katz, 2003).

General Procedures
- Use an iced lemon glycerine swab to perform the thermal-tactile stimulation.
- Instruct the patient to open the mouth.
- Place the iced lemon glycerin swab in the patient's mouth at the base of the anterior faucial pillars.
- Rub the right anterior faucial pillar up and down in a vertical movement.
- Repeat this strategy five times on the right side.
- Repeat this procedure on the left side on the anterior faucial pillar five times.
- Give the patient food or liquids (if using thermal-tactile stimulation as a compensatory strategy).
- Repeat three or four times daily for 5 to 10 minutes each time.

Potential Benefits of This Exercise/Strategy
- Increased stimulation in the oral cavity
- Increased sensory awareness
- Increased initiation of the swallow reflex

Protocol for Thermal-Tactile Stimulation Exercise/Strategy: *Explanation and Instruction to the Patient*		
	Explanation in English	**Explicación en Español**
Clinician	This Thermal-Tactile Stimulation exercise/strategy helps to improve the initiation of your swallow. This exercise/strategy may help you to increase the speed of your swallow.	Este ejercicio/estrategia de Estímulo Táctil le ayuda a mejorar la iniciación de su tragar. Este ejercicio/estrategia le puede ayudar a aumentar la velocidad de su tragar.
	Instruction in English	**Instrucción en Español**
Clinician	1. I will place an iced swab in your mouth. 2. I will rub the iced swab on the right and left sides of the back of your throat. 3. Please open your mouth and keep it open. 4. I will repeat this exercise/strategy five times on the right side. 5. I will repeat the same exercise/strategy on the left side. 6. I will give you some food or liquid, and I want you to swallow [if thermal-tactile stimulation is being used as a compensatory strategy].	1. Voy a poner un aplicador helado en su boca. 2. Voy a tallar el aplicador helado en los lados derecho y izquierdo de lo atrás de su garganta. 3. Por favor abra su boca y manténgala abierta. 4. Voy a hacer este ejercicio/estrategia cinco veces en el lado derecho. 5. Voy a repetir la mismo ejercicio/estrategia en el lado izquierdo. 6. Le voy a dar comida o líquido y quiero que trague [si el estímulo táctilse esta usando como estrtegia compensatoria].

Treatment for Pharyngeal Phase Dysphagia
Improving the Initiation of the Pharyngeal Swallow
Protocol 5.3 (English/Spanish)

Suck Swallow Exercise

The *Suck Swallow Exercise* is a set of procedures used to improve the onset of the pharyngeal swallow (Logemann, 1998; Swigert, 2000).

General Procedures
- Instruct the patient to suck the saliva in the mouth with the tongue as hard as possible.
- Tell the patient to squeeze the lips as hard as possible.
- Have the patient swallow.
- Repeat this exercise 10 times.

Potential Benefits of This Exercise
- Increased sensory awareness in the oral cavity
- Decreased delay in the trigger the swallow

Protocol for Suck Swallow Exercise: *Explanation and Instruction to the Patient*		
	Explanation in English	**Explicación en Español**
Clinician	This Suck Swallow Exercise may help you to increase the speed of the initiation of your swallow. This exercise may help your throat when you swallow.	Este ejercicio de Trago de Chupar le ayuda a iniciar su tragar. Este ejercicio le puede ayudar a su garganta cuando trague.
	Instruction in English	**Instrucción en Español**
Clinician	1. Please suck the saliva in your mouth and squeeze your lips as hard as you can. 2. Please swallow. 3. Please repeat this exercise 10 times.	1. Por favor chupe la saliva en su boca y apriete sus labios lo mas fuerte que pueda. 2. Por favor trague. 3. Por favor repita este ejercicio 10 veces.

Treatment for Pharyngeal Phase Dysphagia
Improving the Initiation of the Pharyngeal Swallow
Protocol 5.4 (English/Spanish)

Textured Bolus Strategy

The *Textured Bolus Strategy* is a set of procedures used to increase sensation when the trigger of the pharyngeal swallow reflex is delayed or absent (Perlman. 1993; Swigert, 2000).

General Procedures

- Present a teaspoon of tapioca, pudding, or rice pudding to the patient.
- Repeat for five trials, or as many as the patient can tolerate.

Note to the Clinician

- Use clinical judgement when deciding to implement this strategy into the patient's therapy program.
- The patient should be safe on pureed or pudding food consistencies before implementing this compensatory strategy.

Potential Benefits of This Strategy

- Increased oral sensory awareness.
- Increased trigger of the pharyngeal swallow.

Protocol for Textured Bolus Strategy: *Explanation and Instruction to the Patient*		
	Explanation in English	**Explicación en Español**
Clinician	This Textured Bolus Strategy helps to increase the sensation in your tongue and throat. This strategy may prevent food or liquid from falling into your throat or airway.	Esta Estrategia de Bolo con Textura le ayuda a aumentar la sensación en su lengua y garganta. Esta estrategia le puede ayudar a evitar que entre comida o líquidos a la garganta o vía respiratoria.
	Instruction in English	**Instrucción en Español**
Clinician	1. I will put a teaspoon in your mouth with pudding/tapioca/rice pudding on it. 2. Please open your mouth so that I can put the spoon in your mouth. 3. Please close your lips around the spoon. 4. Please swallow now. 5. I will give you a teaspoon of pudding/tapioca/rice pudding for a total of five times.	1. Voy a ponerle una cuchara con pudín/tapioca/atole de arroz en su boca. 2. Por favor abra su boca para que pueda ponerle la cuchara en su boca. 3. Por favor cierre sus labios alrededor de la cuchara. 4. Por favor trague. 5. Le voy a dar cinco cucharadas de pudín/ tapioca/atole de arroz por un total de cinco veces.

Treatment for Pharyngeal Phase Dysphagia
Improving Initiation of the Pharyngeal Swallow
Protocol 5.5 (English/Spanish)

Sour Bolus Strategy

The *Sour Bolus Strategy* is used to increase sensation when the trigger of the pharyngeal swallow reflex is delayed or absent (Logemann, Pauloski, Colangelo, Lazarus, Fujiu, & Kahrilas, 1995; Swigert, 2000).

General Procedures
- Use regular or thickened citrus juices (e.g., orange juice).
- Present a teaspoon with juice on it.
- Repeat for five trials,, or as many as the patient can tolerate.

Note to the Clinician
- Use clinical judgement when deciding to implement this strategy into the patient's therapy program.
- The patient should be able to safely consume regular or thickened juices before this compensatory stragety is implemented.

Potential Benefits of This Strategy
- Increased oral sensory awareness
- Increased pharyngeal trigger of the swallow

Protocol for Sour Bolus Strategy: *Explanation and Instruction to the Patient*		
	Explanation in English	**Explicación en Español**
Clinician	This Sour Bolus Strategy helps to increase the sensation in your tongue and throat. This strategy may prevent food or liquid from falling into your throat or airway.	Esta Estrategia de Bolo Amargo le ayuda a aumentar la sensación en su lengua y su garganta. Esta estrategia le puede ayudar a evitar que entre comida o líquidos a la garganta o vía respiratoria.
	Instruction in English	**Instrucción en Español**
Clinician	1. I will put a teaspoon of orange juice in your mouth. 2. Please open your mouth so that I can put the spoon in your mouth. 3. Please close your lips around the spoon. 4. Please swallow now. 5. I will give you a teaspoon of orange juice five times.	1. Le voy a poner una cuchara de jugo de naranja en su boca. 2. Por favor abra su boca para que le pueda meter la cuchara en su boca. 3. Por favor cierre los labios alrededor de la cuchara. 4. Por favor trague. 5. Le voy a dar cucharadas de jugo de naranja cinco veces.

Treatment for Pharyngeal Phase Dysphagia
Improving Initiation of the Pharyngeal Swallow
Protocol 5.6 (English/Spanish)

Cold Bolus Strategy

The *Cold Bolus Strategy* is a set of procedures used to increase sensation when the trigger of the pharyngeal swallow reflex is delayed or absent (Logemann, 1998; Murry & Carrau, 2006; Swigert, 2000).

General Procedures

- Present one teaspoon of applesauce or pudding that is really cold.
- Give the patient as many trials as the patient tolerates without signs or symptoms of aspiration.

Note to the Clinician

- Do not use ice cream or frozen yogurt for the cold bolus. Ice cream and frozen yogurt melt once they get inside the mouth and turn into a thinner consistency.
- Use clinical judgement when deciding to include this strategy.
- The patient should be able to safely ingest food of pureed consistency before implementation of this compensatory strategy.

Potential Benefits of This Strategy

- Increased oral sensory awareness
- Increased trigger of the pharyngeal swallow

Protocol for Cold Bolus Strategy: *Explanation and Instruction to the Patient*		
	Explanation in English	**Explicación en Español**
Clinician	This Cold Bolus Strategy helps to increase the sensation in your tongue and throat. This strategy may prevent food or liquid from falling into your throat or airway.	Esta Estrategia de Bolo Frió le ayuda a aumentar la sensación en su lengua y su garganta. Esta estrategia le puede ayudar a evitar que entre comida o líquidos a la garganta o vía repiratoria.
	Instruction in English	**Instrucción en Español**
Clinician	1. I will put a spoon with cold applesauce/pudding in your mouth. 2. The applesauce/pudding is going to be very cold. 3. Please swallow. 4. I will give you a teaspoon with cold applesauce/pudding five times.	1. Voy a ponerle una cuchara con puré de manzana/pudín frió en su boca. 2. El puré de manzana/pudín va estar muy frió. 3. Por favor trague. 4. Le voy a dar cucharadas con puré de manzana /pudín frió cinco veces.

Treatment for Pharyngeal Phase Dysphagia
Improving Initiation of the Pharyngeal Swallow
Protocol 5.7 (English/Spanish)

Small Bolus Strategy

The *Small Bolus Strategy* is a set of procedures used with patients that exhibit delayed initiation of the pharyngeal swallow (Lazarus, Logemann, Rademaker, Kahrilas, Pajak, Lazar, et al., 1993; Swigert, 2000).

General Procedures
- Instruct the patient or caregiver to use a teaspoon or pediatric spoon to ingest food and liquids.
- Control the amount of food or liquid that goes into the patient's mouth.
- Tell the patient or caregiver how much food or liquid should be placed on the teaspoon (this amount will vary from patient to patient).
- Use clinical judgement when deciding how much food or liquid should go on the teaspoon or pediatric spoon.

Note to the Clinician
- Use clinical judgement when deciding to implement this strategy into the patient's therapy program.
- Make sure that the patient is not at risk for aspiration when implementing this strategy.

Potential Benefits of This Strategy
- Increased control of the bolus
- Decreased risk for aspiration and choking

Protocol for Small Bolus Strategy: *Explanation and Instruction to the Patient*		
	Explanation in English	**Explicación en Español**
Clinician	This Small Bolus Strategy helps to increase the sensation in your tongue and throat. This strategy may prevent food or liquids from falling into your throat or airway.	Esta Estrategia de Bolo Chico le ayuda a aumentar la sensación en su lengua y su garganta. Esta estrategia le puede ayudar a evitar que entre comida o líquidos a la garganta o a la vía respiratoria.
	Instruction in English	**Instrucción en Español**
Clinician	1. Please use a teaspoon or small spoon to eat with. 2. I will show you how much food or liquid I want you to put on your spoon every time you swallow. 3. This is the kind of spoon I want you to use and this is the amount of food and liquid I want you to put on the spoon every time you put food or liquid in your mouth.	1. Por favor use una cuchara o cucharilla para comer. 2. Le voy a enseñar que tanta comida o líquido quiero que ponga en la cuchara cada vez que traga. 3. Esta es la clase de cuchara que quiero que use y esta es la cantidad de comida o líquido que quiero que ponga en la cuchara cada vez que se ponga comida o líquido en su boca.

Treatment for Pharyngeal Phase Dysphagia
Reducing Residue in the Valleculae

Overview

Many patients with pharyngeal phase dysphagia have decreased tongue base movement and decreased posterior pharyngeal wall movement. As a result, the base of the tongue and the posterior pharyngeal wall may not contact each other. This can result in residue in the valleculae. The patient is at risk for aspiration when this occurs. This section outlines rehabilitative swallow therapy exercises/strategies and compensatory swallow therapy exercises that will decrease the occurrence of residue in the valleculae (Logemann, 1998; Murry & Carrau, 2006):

Rehabilitative Swallow Therapy Exercises/Strategies

The following rehabilitative swallow therapy exercises/strategies are described next:

- Effortful Swallow Exercise/Strategy
- Mendelsohn Maneuver Exercise/Strategy
- Modified Tongue Anchor Exercise
- Supraglottic Swallow Strategy
- Lying Down on the Side Strategy

Compensatory Swallow Therapy Exercises

The following compensatory strategies also are described:

- /k/ Productions Exercise
- Dry Gargle Exercise
- Big Yawn Exercise

Treatment for Pharyngeal Phase Dysphagia
Reducing Residue in the Valleculae
Protocol 5.8 (English/Spanish)

Effortful Swallow Exercise/Strategy

The *Effortful Swallow Exercise/Strategy* is a set of procedures used to decrease residue in the valleculae (Kahrilas, Logemann, Lin, & Ergun, 1992; Pounderoux & Kahrilas, 1995; Swigert, 2000).

General Procedures
- Instruct the patient to put some food or liquid inside the mouth.
- Tell the patient to squeeze and push the tongue backward as much as possible while swallowing (Swigert, 2000).
- The patient uses this strategy during mealtimes.

Note to the Clinician
- Use clinical judgement when deciding to implement this exercise/strategy into the patient's therapy program.
- Make sure that the patient is not at risk for aspiration before implementing this exercise/strategy.

Potential Benefits of This Exercise/Strategy
- Increased tongue base strength
- Increased tongue base control
- Decreased residue in the valleculae

Protocol for Effortful Swallow Exercise/Strategy: *Explanation and Instruction to the Patient*		
	Explanation in English	**Explicación en Español**
Clinician	This Effortful Swallow Exercise/Strategy helps to increase the strength in the back of your tongue and throat. This exercise/strategy may prevent food or liquids from getting stuck in your throat.	Este Ejercicio/Estrategia de Trago con Esfuerzo le ayuda a aumentar la fuerza en lo de atrás de su lengua y su garganta. Este ejercicio/estrategia puede ayudarle a evitar que la comida o líquidos se atoren en su garganta.
	Instruction in English	**Instrucción en Español**
Clinician	1. Please place some food or liquid into your mouth. 2. Please chew your food [if the patient's diet includes foods that require chewing]. 3. Please push and squeeze your tongue backward as hard as you can while you swallow. 4. Please complete this exercise/strategy every time you put food or liquid into your mouth.	1. Por favor ponga comida o líquido en su boca. 2. Por favor mastique su comida [si la dieta del paciente incluye comidas que requieren ser masticadas]. 3. Por favor empuje y aplane su lengua hacia atrás lo mas fuerte que pueda mientras que traga. 4. Por favor haga esta estrategia/ejercicio cada vez que se ponga comida o líquido en su boca.

Treatment for Pharyngeal Phase Dysphagia
Reducing Residue in the Valleculae
Protocol 5.9 (English/Spanish)

Mendelsohn Maneuver Exercise/Strategy

The *Mendelsohn Maneuver Exercise/Strategy* is a set of procedures used to decrease residue in the valleculae (Bartolome & Neuman, 1993; Ding, Larson, Logemann, & Rademaker, 2002; Logemann, Kahrilas, Cheng, Pauloski, Gibbons, Rademaker, & Lin, 1992).

General Procedures
- Instruct the patient to put a hand on the larynx (do not have the patient hold the larynx).
- Tell the patient to swallow (if using the Mendelsohn maneuver as a strategy, the clinician should present food or liquids).
- Show the patient when the larynx elevates.
- Instruct the patient to swallow, and then have the patient identify the highest point when the larynx is elevated.
- Repeat this exercise five times.
- Instruct the patient to put the hand on the larynx and swallow.
- Have the patient identify the highest point of the swallow and squeeze the muscles in the back of the tongue as hard and as long as possible without letting the larynx come back down.
- Repeat this exercise/strategy 10 times.

Note to the Clinician
- Initially, this is done as an exercise/strategy and then implemented as a compensatory strategy when the patient is eating.

Potential Benefits of This Exercise/Strategy
- Increased tongue base control
- Decreased premature spillage of the bolus into the pharynx
- Decreased residue in the valleculae

Protocol for Mendelsohn Maneuver Exercise/Strategy: *Explanation and Instruction to the Patient*		
	Explanation in English	**Explicación en Español**
Clinician	This Mendelsohn Maneuver Strategy/ Exercise helps to move your throat muscles up. This strategy/exercise may prevent food or liquids from getting stuck in your throat.	Esta Eatrategia/Ejercicio de Maniobra Mendelsohn le ayuda a mover los músculos de su garganta para arriba. Esta estrategia/ejercicio puede ayudarle a evitar que la comida o los líquidos se atoren en la garganta.
	Instruction in English	**Instrucción en Español**
Clinician	1. Please put your hand on your throat. 2. I will put some food in your mouth [if the Mendelsohn maneuver is being used as a compensatory strategy]. 3. Please swallow and feel your larynx go up. 4. Please show me with your hand where the larynx goes up the highest. 5. Please swallow when your larynx reaches the highest point. 6. Please squeeze the back muscles of your tongue for as long and as hard as you can without letting your larynx go down. 7. Please repeat this exercise/strategy five times.	1. Por favor ponga su mano en su garganta. 2. Voy a poner comida en su boca [si estan usando el manobria mendelsohn como estrategia compensatgoria. 3. Por favor trague y sienta su laringe cuando se mueve para arriba. 4. Por favor enséñeme con su mano donde la laringe se alza lo mas alto. 5. Por favor trague cuando su laringe llegue al punto mas alto. 6. Quiero que apriete los músculos de atrás de su lengua lo mas largo y fuerte que pueda sin dejar ir la laringe para abajo. 7. Por favor repita esta estrategia/ ejercicio cinco veces.

Treatment for Pharyngeal Phase Dysphagia
Reducing Residue in the Valleculae
Protocol 5.10 (English/Spanish)

Modified Tongue Anchor Exercise

The *Modified Tongue Anchor Exercise* is a set of procedures used to decrease residue in the valleculae (Fujiu & Logemann, 1996; Lazarus, Logemann, Song, Rademaker, & Kahrilas, 2002; Murry & Carrau, 2006).

General Procedures
- Instruct the patient to stick out the tongue outside of the mouth.
- Have the patient gently hold onto the tongue with the teeth.
- Tell the patient to swallow while holding onto the tongue with the teeth.
- Repeat this exercise 10 times.

Potential Benefits of This Exercise
- Increased tongue base control
- Increased tongue base strength
- Decreased residue in the valleculae

Protocol for Modified Tongue Anchor Exercise: *Explanation and Instruction to the Patient*		
	Explanation in English	**Explicación en Español**
Clinician	This Modified Tongue Anchor exercise helps to strengthen the walls of your throat. This exercise may prevent food or liquids from getting stuck in your throat.	Este ejercicio modificado de Anclar la Lengua le ayuda a reforzar las paredes de su garganta. Este ejercicio puede ayudarle a evitar que la comida o los líquidos se atoren en su garganta.
	Instruction in English	**Instrucción en Español**
Clinician	1. Please stick the front part of your tongue outside of the mouth. 2. Please bite down gently on your tongue. 3. Please continue to hold your tongue and swallow. 4. Please repeat this exercise 10 times.	1. Por favor saque la parte de enfrente de su lengua fuera de su boca. 2. Por favor muerda su lengua suavemente. 3. Por favor continué deteniendo su lengua y trague. 4. Por favor repita este ejercicio 10 veces.

Treatment for Pharyngeal Phase Dysphagia
Reducing Residue in the Valleculae
Protocol 5.11 (English/Spanish)

Supraglottic Swallow Exercise/Strategy

The *Supraglottic Swallow Exercise/Strategy* is a set of procedures used to reduce residue in the valleculae (Bulow, Olsson, & Ekberg, 2001; Kahrilas, Logemann, & Gibbons, 1992; Logemann & Kahrilas, 1990; Singh, Brockbank, Frost, & Tyler, 1995; Swigert, 2000).

General Procedures
- Utilize this strategy without presentation of food and then introduce food while incorporating this exercise/strategy.
- Tell the patient to take a deep breath and then exhale a little bit of air out.
- Instruct the patient to hold the rest of the breath.
- Place food or liquid into the oral cavity (the patient should still be holding the breath).
- Instruct the patient to swallow while continuing to hold the breath during the swallow.
- Tell the patient to cough immediately after the swallow.
- Instruct the patient to swallow again.

Note to the Clinician
- Use clinical judgement when deciding to implement this exercise/strategy into the patient's therapy program.
- Make sure that the patient is not at risk for aspiration before implementing this exercise/strategy.

Potential Benefits of This Exercise/Strategy
- Increased laryngeal closure in case premature spillage occurs
- Decreased residue in the valleculae
- Decreased risk for aspiration

Protocol for Supraglottic Swallow Exercise/Strategy: *Explanation and Instruction to the Patient*		
	Explanation in English	**Explicacion en Español**
Clinician	This Supraglottic Swallow Exercise/Strategy helps to protect the airway before and during the swallow. This exercise/strategy may assure that food or liquid does not get stuck in your throat.	Este Ejercicio/Estrategia de Trago Supraglotticle ayuda a proteger la vía aérea antes y durante el trago. Este ejercicio/ estrategia le asegurar que comida o líquidos no se atoren en su garganta.
	Instruction in English	**Instrucción en Español**
Clinician	1. Please take a deep breath and then exhale a little bit of air out. 2. Please hold in the rest of the air and don't let go of it. 3. I will put some food in your mouth. 4. Please continue holding your breath while you swallow your food. 5. Please cough [once the patient finishes swallowing the food]. 6. Please swallow again.	1. Por favor respire profundamente para adentro y luego respire poco del aire para afuera. 2. Por favor detenga el resto del aire y no lo deje ir. 3. Le voy a poner comida en su boca. 4. Por favor continué deteniendo la respiración mientras que traga su comida. 5. Por favor tosa. 6. Por favor trague otra vez.

Treatment for Pharyngeal Phase Dysphagia
Reducing Residue in the Valleculae
Protocol 5.12 (English/Spanish)

Lying Down on the Side Strategy

The *Lying Down on the Side Strategy* is a set of procedures used to reduce unilateral residue in the valleculae (Drake, O'Donoghue, Bartram, Lindsey, & Greenwood, 1997; Rasley, Logemann, Kahrilas, Rademaker, Pauloski, & Dodds, 1993).

General Procedures
- Instruct the patient to lie down or tilt the head toward the strong side (the side without residue).
- Place a pillow behind the neck and position it securely.
- Present one trial of food to the patient.
- Tell the patient to swallow.
- Implement this strategy during mealtimes.

Note to the Clinician
- The patient's head should be supported.

Potential Benefits of This Strategy
- Increased flow of food/liquid through the pharynx
- Decreased residue in the valleculae

Protocol for Lying Down on the Side Strategy: *Explanation and Instruction to the Patient*		
	Explanation in English	**Explanación en Español**
Clinician	This Lying Down on the Side Strategy helps to decrease the risk of aspiration. This strategy may help you reduce the amount of food and liquid that gets stuck in your throat.	Esta Estrategia de Tendido en el Lado le ayuda a disminuir el riesgo de aspiracion. Esta estrategia puede ayudarle a reducir la cantidad de comida o líquido que se atora en su garganta.
	Instruction in English	**Instrucción en Español**
Clinician	1. Please lie down on your right/left side. 2. I will put a pillow under your head. 3. I will give you some food/liquid to swallow. 4. Please use this strategy at every mealtime.	1. Por favor acuéstese en su lado derecho/izquierdo. 2. Voy a ponerle una almohada bajo su cabeza. 3. Voy a darle comida/líquido para que trague. 4. Por favor use esta estrategia cada vez que coma o tome.

Treatment for Pharyngeal Phase Dysphagia
Reducing Residue in the Valleculae
Protocol 5.13 (English/Spanish)

/k/ Tongue Production Exercise

The */k/ Tongue Production Exercise* is a set of procedures used to decrease the residue in the valleculae (Murry & Carrau, 2006; Swigert, 2000).

General Procedures
- Provide a list of words to the patient.
- Instruct the patient to produce words with stress on the beginning phoneme /k/.
- Complete one list of words two times.

Note to the Clinician
- Check to see if the patient wears corrective lenses for vision before giving the patient the list.
- Say the word and then have the patient repeat the same word if the patient has visual impairments.

Potential Benefits of This Exercise
- Increased back of tongue control and strength
- Decreased residue in the valleculae after the swallow

Protocol for /k/ Tongue Production Exercise: *Explanation and Instruction to the Patient*		
	Explanation in English	**Explicación en Español**
Clinician	This /k/ Tongue Production exercise helps to increase the strength in the back of your tongue and throat. This exercise may help to prevent food or liquids from getting stuck in your throat.	Este ejercicio de La Lengua en Producción de /k/ le ayuda a aumentar la fuerza en lo de atrás de su lengua y su garganta. Este ejercicio le puede ayudar a evitar que la comida o los líquidos se atoren en su garganta.
	Instruction in English	**Instrucción en Español**
Clinician	1. I will give you a list of words and I will say some words to you. 2. Please read them aloud and repeat the same words that I say. 3. When you say the words, please put emphasis on the beginning sound which will be /k/. 4. Please repeat one list of words two times.	1. Le voy a dar una lista de palabras y le voy a decir algunas palabras. 2. Por favor las lee en voz alta y repita las mismas palabras que yo diga. 3. Cuando digan las palabras quiero que ponga énfasis en el sonido inicial que será /k/. 4. Por favor repita la lista de palabras dos veces.

/k/ Word List in English

1. cab	16. cash	31. key
2. calm	17. call	32. cough
3. cane	18. can	33. cart
4. car	19. cape	34. cane
5. case	20. cut	35. cod
6. coast	21. kite	36. cone
7. cold	22. cup	37. cop
8. cook	23. coal	38. college
9. corn	24. coat	39. copy
10. collar	25. comb	40. cub
11. count	26. cool	41. king
12. cage	27. color	42. kind
13. came	28. cookie	43. cat
14. cans	29. court	44. cow
15. care	30. kick	45. core

/k/ Word List in Spanish

1. cabra	16. cueva	31. cambiar
2. caja	17. calle	32. cadera
3. karate	18. carta	33. caro
4. coco	19. cachete	34. casa
5. cala	20. calor	35. caer
6. cuento	21. cama	36. caber
7. carro	22. caída	37. camino
8. callo	23. cabello	38. casar
9. café	24. caballo	39. caso
10. costo	25. cada	40. cabeza
11. calcetín	26. cabaña	41. causa
12. kilo	27. cámara	42. cara
13. calma	28. con	43. cazo
14. calcular	29. camello	44. coma
15. cantar	30. cargo	45. comer

Treatment for Pharyngeal Phase Dysphagia
Reducing Residue in the Valleculae
Protocol 5.14 (English/Spanish)

Dry Gargle Exercise

The *Dry Gargle Exercise* is a set of procedures used to decrease the residue in the valleculae (Logemann, 1998).

General Procedures
- Instruct the patient to pretend to be gargling water or mouthwash.
- Have the patient pretend to gargle for 5 seconds.
- Repeat this exercise 10 times.

Note to the Clinician
- Do not present any water or mouthwash to the patient for this exercise.

Potential Benefits of This Exercise
- Increased tongue base control
- Increased tongue base strength
- Decreased residue in the valleculae

Protocol for Dry Gargle Exercise: *Explanation and Instruction to the Patient*		
	Explanation in English	**Explicación en Español**
Clinician	This Dry Gargle Exercise helps to increase the strength in the back of your tongue and throat. This exercise may help you reduce the amount of food and liquid that gets stuck in your throat after you swallow.	Este Ejercicio de Gárgara Seca le ayuda a aumentar la fuerza en lo de atrás de su lengua y su garganta. Este ejercicio puede ayudarle a reducir la cantidad de comida o líquido que se atora en su garganta después de que traga.
	Instruction in English	**Instrucción en Español**
Clinician	1. Please pretend that you are gargling mouthwash or water. 2. Please gargle for 5 seconds. 3. Please repeat this exercise 10 times.	1. Por favor pretenda que esta gargarizando con enjuague de boca o agua. 2. Por favor gargaricé por 5 segundos. 3. Por favor repita este ejercicio 10 veces.

Treatment for Pharyngeal Phase Dysphagia
Reducing Residue in the Valleculae
Protocol 5.15 (English/Spanish)

Big Yawn Exercise

The *Big Yawn Exercise* is a set of procedures used to reduce residue in the valleculae (Logemann, 1998).

General Procedures
- Instruct the patient to yawn as wide as possible (this exercise will facilitate the upward movement of the base of the tongue).
- Ask the patient to hold the yawn for 2 seconds.
- Repeat this exercise five times.

Potential Benefits of This Exercise
- Increased tongue base control
- Increased tongue base strength
- Decreased residue in the valleculae

Protocol for Big Yawn Exercise: *Explanation and Instruction to the Patient*		
	Explanation in English	**Explicación en Español**
Clinician	This Big Yawn Exercise helps to increase the strength in the back of your tongue and throat. This exercise may prevent food or liquids from getting stuck in your throat.	Este ejercicio de Bostezo Grande le ayuda a aumentar la fuerza en lo de atrás de su lengua y su garganta. Este ejercicio le puede ayudar a reducir la cantidad de comida o líquido que se atora en su garganta.
	Instruction in English	**Instrucción en Español**
Clinician	1. Please yawn as wide as possible.	1. Por favor bostéce lo más ancho posible.
	2. Please keep yawning for 2 seconds.	2. Por favor manténgase bosteceando por 2 segundos.
	3. Please repeat this exercise five times.	3. Por favor repita este ejercicio cinco veces.

Treatment for Pharyngeal Phase Dysphagia
Reducing the Residue in the Pharynx

Overview

Patients with pharyngeal phase dysphagia may exhibit pharyngeal residue. This problem may be secondary to reduced pharyngeal wall contraction.

This section presents rehabilitative swallow therapy exercise/strategies that can be used to decrease residue in the pharynx (Logemann, 1998; Murry & Carrau, 2006).

Rehabilitative Swallow Therapy Exercise/Strategies

The following rehabilitative swallow therapy exercise/strategies are described next:

- Tongue Anchor Exercise
- Lying Down on the Side Strategy
- Head Turn Exercise/Strategy
- Head Tilt Strategy

Treatment for Pharyngeal Phase Dysphagia
Reducing Residue in the Pharynx
Protocol 5.16 (English/Spanish)

Tongue Anchor Exercise

The *Tongue Anchor Exercise* is a set of procedures used to decrease residue in the pharynx (Logemann, 1998; Swigert, 2000).

General Procedures
- Instruct the patient to stick out the tongue outside of the mouth.
- Have the patient gently hold onto the tongue with the teeth.
- Tell the patient to swallow while holding onto the tongue with the teeth.
- Repeat this exercise 10 times.

Potential Benefits of This Exercise
- Increased pharyngeal wall pressure
- Decreased residue in the pharynx

Protocol for Tongue Anchor Exercise: *Explanation and Instruction to the Patient*		
	Explanation in English	**Explicación en Español**
Clinician	This Tongue Anchor Exercise helps to strengthen your throat. This exercise may prevent food or liquids from getting stuck in your throat.	Este Ejercicio de Anclar la Lengua le ayuda a refozar su garganta. Este ejercicio puede ayudarle a evitar que la comida o los líquidos se atoren en su garganta.
	Instruction in English	**Instrucción en Español**
Clinician	1. Please stick the front part of your tongue outside of the mouth. 2. Please gently bite down on your tongue. 3. Please continue holding your tongue and swallow. 4. Please repeat this exercise 10 times.	1. Por favor saque la parte de enfrente de su lengua fuera de su boca. 2. Por favor muerda su lengua suavemente. 3. Por favor continué deteniendo su lengua y trague. 4. Por favor repita este ejercicio 10 veces.

Treatment for Pharyngeal Phase Dysphagia
Reducing Residue in the Pharynx
Protocol 5.17 (English/Spanish)

Lying Down on the Side Strategy

The *Lying Down on the Side Strategy* is a set of procedures used to reduce unilateral residue in the pharynx (Drake, O'Donoghue, Bartram, Lindsey, & Greenwood, 1997; Rasley, Logemann, Kahrilas, Rademaker, Pauloski, & Dodds, 1993).

General Procedures
- Instruct the patient to lie down on the unaffected side (the side without residue) or to tilt the head toward that side.
- Place a pillow behind the neck and position it securely.
- Present one trial of food to the patient.
- Tell the patient to swallow.
- Implement this strategy during meal times.

Note to the Clinician
- The patient's head should be supported.

Potential Benefits of This Strategy
- Decreased residue in the pharynx
- Decreased risk for aspiration

Protocol for Lying Down on the Side Strategy: *Explanation and Instruction to the Patient*		
	Explanation in English	**Explicación en Español**
Clinician	This Lying Down on the Side Strategy helps to strengthen your throat. This exercise may help you reduce the amount of food and liquid that gets stuck in your throat.	Esta estrategia de Tendido en el Lado le ayuda a refozar su garganta. Este ejercicio puede ayudarle a reducir la cantidad de comida o líquido que se atora en su garganta.
	Instruction in English	**Instrucción en Español**
Clinician	1. Please lie down on your right/left side. 2. I will put a pillow under your head. 3. I will give you some food/liquid to swallow. 4. Please use this strategy at every mealtime.	1. Por favor acuéstese en su lado derecho/izquierdo. 2. Voy a ponerle una almohada bajo su cabeza. 3. Voy a darle comida/líquido para que trague. 4. Por favor use esta estrategia cada vez que come o tome.

Treatment for Pharyngeal Phase Dysphagia
Reducing Residue in the Pharynx
Protocol 5.18 (English/Spanish)
Head Turn Exercise/Strategy

The *Head Turn Exercise/Strategy* is a set of procedures used to reduce pharyngeal residue (Logemann, Kahrilas, Kobara, & Vakil, 1989; Logemann & Kahrilas, 1990; Rasley, Logemann, Kahrilas, Rademaker, Pauloski, & Dodds, 1993; Silbergleit, Waring, Sullivan, & Maynard, 1991).

General Procedures
- Instruct the patient to turn the head all the way to the right/left side (whichever side is more affected).
- Present food to the patient and ask the patient to swallow.
- Implement this strategy during the patient's therapeutic feedings.

Potential Benefits of This Exercise/Strategy
- Decreased pharyngeal residue
- Decreased risk for aspiration

Protocol for Head Turn Exercise/Strategy: *Explanation and Instruction to the Patient*		
	Explanation in English	**Explicación en Español**
Clinician	This Head Turn Exercise/Strategy helps to strengthen the throat muscles on the strong side of your throat. This exercise/strategy may help the food or liquids to go down the way they should.	Este Ejercicio/Estrategia de Voltear la Cabeza le ayuda a reforzar los músculos de los lados fuertes de su garganta. Este ejercicio/estrategia puede ayudar a que los líquidos y la comida se vayan a donde deben ir.
	Instruction in English	**Instrucción en Español**
Clinician	1. Please sit up straight in your chair. 2. Please turn your head all the way to the left/right side. 3. Please swallow the food that I give you with your head turned completely to the right/left side. 4. Please continue this exercise/ strategy throughout your meals.	1. Por favor siéntese derecho en su silla. 2. Por favor voltee su cabeza todo lo que se pueda al lado izquierdo/ derecho. 3. Por favor trague la comida que le doy con su cabeza volteada al lado derecho/izquierdo. 4. Por favor continué este ejercicio/ estrategia durante sus comidas.

Treatment for Pharyngeal Phase Dysphagia
Reducing the Residue in the Pharynx
Protocol 5.19 (English/Spanish)

Head Tilt Strategy

The *Head Tilt Strategy* is used to reduce unilateral pharyngeal residue (Logemann, 1998; Singh, Brockbank, Frost, & Tyler, 1995).

General Procedures

- Make sure the patient is on the safest oral diet when the clinician implements this compensatory strategy.
- Have the patient place food in the mouth.
- Tell the patient to tilt the head to the right/left side (whichever side is the strongest).
- Instruct the patient to swallow once the head is tilted.
- Remind the patient to do this strategy every time that food is placed inside the mouth.

Potential Benefits of This Strategy

- Decreased pharyngeal residue
- Decreased risk for aspiration

Protocol for Head Tilt Strategy: *Explanation and Instruction to the Patient*		
	Explanation in English	**Explicación en Español**
Clinician	This Head Tilt Strategy helps strengthen the throat muscles. This strategy may help to make sure that food or liquid does not get stuck inside your throat.	Esta Estrategia de Inclinar la Cabeza le ayuda a reforzar los músculos de la garganta. Esta estrategia le puede ayudar asegurar que la comida o los líquidos no se atoren en su garganta.
	Instruction in English	**Instrucción en Español**
Clinician	1. Please put the food or liquid in your mouth. 2. Please tilt your head to the left/right side [whichever side is the stronger]. 3. Please swallow your food/liquid once your head is tilted. 4. Please do this strategy every time you put food or liquid in your mouth.	1. Por favor ponga la comida o el líquido en su boca. 2. Por favor incline su cabeza al (lado izquierdo/derecho [cuál sea el más fuerte]. 3. Por favor trague su comida/líquido cuando su cabeza esta inclinada. 4. Por favor haga esta estrategia cada vez que se pone comida o líquido en su boca.

Treatment for Pharyngeal Phase Dysphagia
Increasing Laryngeal Closure

Overview

Patients with pharyngeal phase dysphagia may have difficulty achieving laryngeal closure of the airway. As a result, these patients are at risk for aspiration. The following section outlines compensatory swallow therapy exercises and rehabilitative swallow therapy exercise/strategies that can be used with patients who exhibit decreased laryngeal closure (Logemann, 1998; Murry & Carrau, 2006).

Compensatory Swallow Therapy Exercises

The following compensatory swallow therapy exercises are described next:

- Pulling Exercise
- Pushing Exercise

Rehabilitative Swallow Therapy Exercise/Strategies

The following rehabilitative swallow therapy exercises/strategies also are described:

- Valsalva Maneuver Exercise
- Super-Supraglottic Swallow Exercise/Strategy
- Supraglottic Swallow Exercise/Strategy
- Chin Down Exercise/Strategy
- Head Turn Exercise/Strategy
- Head Turn with Chin Down Exercise/Strategy

Treatment for Pharyngeal Phase Dysphagia
Increasing Laryngeal Closure
Protocol 5.20 (English/Spanish)

Pulling Exercise

The *Pulling Exercise* is a set of procedures used to increase laryngeal closure (Swigert, 2000).

General Procedures
- Instruct the patient to place the hands in the clinician's hands.
- Tell the patient to pull on the clinician's hands as hard as possible.
- Repeat this exercise 10 times.
- Instruct the patient to do this procedure and add the production /i/ or /a/ while pulling against the clinician's hands.
- Repeat this exercise 10 times.

Potential Benefits of This Exercise
- Increased laryngeal closure
- Decreased risk for aspiration

Protocol for Pulling Exercise: *Explanation and Instruction to the Patient*		
	Explanation in English	**Explicación en Español**
Clinician	This Pulling Exercise helps to close the airway when you swallow. This exercise may help you to keep food and liquid out of your lungs.	Este Ejercicio de Tirón le ayuda a cerrar la vía aérea. Este ejercicio puede ayudarle a mantener que la comida o los líquidos no entren a su garganta o pulmones.
	Instruction in English	**Instrucción en Español**
Clinician	1. Please sit up straight in your chair.	1. Por favor siéntese derecho en una silla.
	2. I will sit directly in front of you.	2. Me voy a sentar en una silla frente a usted.
	3. Please grab hold of my hands and pull as hard as you can.	3. Por favor agarre mis manos en sus manos y estire lo mas fuerte que pueda.
	4. I will give some resistance.	4. Le voy a dar resistencia.
	5. Please repeat this exercise 10 times.	5. Por favor repita este ejercicio 10 veces.
	6. Please do the same exercise as the one we just did, except when you pull against my hand, I want you to say /i/ and /a/ as you are pulling against my hands.	6. Por favor haga el ejercicio que le enseñe, pero mientras que estira contra mi mano quiero que diga /i/ y /a/ al mismo tiempo que estira mi mano.
	7. Please repeat this exercise 10 times.	7. Por favor repita este ejercicio 10 veces.

Treatment for Pharyngeal Phase Dysphagia
Increasing Laryngeal Closure
Protocol 5.21 (English/Spanish)

Pushing Exercise

The *Pushing Exercise* is a set of procedures used to increase laryngeal closure (Swigert, 2000).

General Procedures

- Instruct the patient to push with the hands against the clinician's hands as hard as possible.
- Repeat this exercise 10 times.
- Have the patient repeat this procedure, except that the patient should vocalize /i/ and /a/ while pushing against the clinician's hands.
- Repeat this exercise 10 times.

Potential Benefits of This Exercise

- Increased laryngeal closure
- Decreased risk for aspiration

Protocol for Pushing Exercise: *Explanation and Instruction to the Patient*		
	Explanation in English	**Explicación en Español**
Clinician	This Pushing Exercise helps to close the airway when you swallow. This exercise may help you to keep food and liquid out of your lungs.	Este Ejercicio de Empujón le ayuda a cerrar la vía aérea . Este ejercicio puede ayudarle a mantener que la comida o líquidos no entren a su garganta o pulmones.
	Instruction in English	**Instrucción en Español**
Clinician	1. Please push against my hands with your hands as hard as you can, for 3 seconds. 2. Please do this exercise 10 times. 3. Please do the same exercise, except that I want you to say /i/ or /a/ when you are pushing against my hands. 4. Please continue pushing and saying /i/ or /a/ for 3 seconds and then relax. 5. Please repeat this exercise 10 times.	1. Por favor empuje contra mis manos con sus manos lo mas fuerte que pueda, por 3 segundos. 2. Por favor haga este ejercicio 10 veces. 3. Por favor haga el mismo ejercicio, pero, quiero que diga /i/ y /a/ mientras que esta empujando contra mis manos. 4. Por favor continué empujando y diciendo /i/ y /a/ por 3 segundos y luego descanse. 5. Por favor repita este ejercicio 10 veces.

Treatment for Pharyngeal Phase Dysphagia
Increasing Laryngeal Closure
Protocol 5.22 (English/Spanish)

Valsalva Maneuver Exercise

The *Valsalva Maneuver Exercise* is a set of procedures used to increase laryngeal closure (McCulloch, Perlman, Palmer, & Van Daele, 1996; Murry & Carrau, 2006; Swigert, 2000).

General Procedures

- Instruct the patient to keep the lips open and to take a deep breath.
- Tell the patient to hold the breath for 3 seconds.
- Repeat this exercise 10 times or as tolerated.

Potential Benefits of This Exercise

- Increased laryngeal closure
- Decreased risk for aspiration

Protocol for Valsalva Maneuver Exercise: *Explanation and Instruction to the Patient*		
	Explanation in English	**Explicación en Español**
Clinician	This Valsalva Maneuver Exercise helps to close the airway when you swallow. This exercise may help you to keep food and liquid out of your lungs.	Este Ejercicio de maniobraVálsala le ayuda a cerrar la vía aérea Este ejercicio puede ayudarle a mantener que la comida o los líquidos no entren a su garganta o pulmones.
	Instruction in English	**Instrucción en Español**
Clinician	1. Please relax. 2. Please leave your lips open. 3. Please take a deep breath and hold it for 3 seconds. 4. Please repeat this exercise 10 times.	1. Por favor descanse. 2. Por favor deje sus labios abiertos. 3. Por favor tome un profundo respiro y deténgalo por 3 segundos. 4. Por favor repita este ejercicio 10 veces.

Treatment for Pharyngeal Phase Dysphagia
Increasing Laryngeal Closure
Protocol 5.23 (English/Spanish)

Super–Supraglottic Swallow Exercise/Strategy

The *Super–Supraglottic Swallow Exercise/Strategy* is a set of procedures used to increase laryngeal closure (Donzelli & Brady, 2004; Kahrilas, Logemann, & Gibbons, 1992; Logemann, Pauloski, Rademaker, & Colangelo, 1997b; Martin, Logemann, Shaker, & Dodds, 1993; Swigert, 2000).

General Procedures
- Implement this exercise/strategy to increase tongue base control on patients who have had a supraglottic laryngectomy (Logemann, 1998).
- Have the patient do this exercise without presentation of food.
- Introduce food while incorporating this strategy.
- Instruct the patient to take a deep breath and then exhale out a small amount of air.
- Tell the patient to hold in the breath as tightly as possible.
- Place food or liquid into the oral cavity (the patient should still be holding the breath).
- Instruct the patient to continue holding the breath while squeezing as hard as possible during the swallow.
- Tell the patient to cough and then swallow again (Swigert, 2000).

Note to the Clinician
- This exercise can be done as a compensatory exercise/strategy with the patient's recommended diet or during treatment.
- Use clinical judgement when deciding to implement this strategy into the patient's therapy program.
- Make sure that the patient is not at risk for aspiration before implementing this strategy.

Potential Benefits of This Exercise/Strategy
- Increased laryngeal closure
- Decreased risk for aspiration

Protocol for Super–Supraglottic Swallow Exercise/Strategy: *Explanation and Instruction to the Patient*		
	Explanation in English	**Explicación en Español**
Clinician	This Super–Supraglottic Swallow Exercise/Strategy helps to close the airway when you swallow. This exercise/strategy may help you to keep food and liquid out of your lungs.	Esta Ejercicio/Estrategia de Trago Súper Supraglottic le ayuda a cerrar la vía aérea. Este ejercicio/estrategia puede ayudarle a mantener que la comida o los líquidos no entren a su garganta o pulmones.
	Instruction in English	**Instrucción en Español**
Clinician	1. Please take a deep breath and then exhale a little bit of air out. 2. Please hold in the rest of the air and don't let go of it. 3. Please put some food in your mouth. 4. Please continue holding your breath and squeeze while you are swallowing your food. 5. Please cough [once the patient finishes swallowing the food]. 6. Please swallow again.	1. Por favor respire y luego deje salir un poco de aire para afuera. 2. Por favor detenga el resto del aire a y no lo deje salir. 3. Por favor póngase comida en su boca. 4. Por favor continué deteniendo su respiración y apriete hacia abajo mientras que traga su comida. 5. Por favor tosa [ya cuando el paciente termine de tragar la comida]. 6. Por favor trague otra vez.

Treatment for Pharyngeal Phase Dysphagia
Increasing Laryngeal Closure
Protocol 5.24 (English/Spanish)

Supraglottic Swallow Exercise/Strategy

The *Supraglottic Swallow Exercise/Strategy* is a set of procedures used to increase laryngeal closure (Bulow, Olsson, & Ekberg, 2001; Kahrilas, Logemann, & Gibbons, 1992; Singh, Brockbank, Frost, & Tyler, 1995; Swigert, 2000).

General Procedures
- Utilize this exercise without presentation of food, and then introduce food while incorporating this strategy.
- Tell the patient to take a deep breath and then exhale a little bit of air out.
- Instruct the patient to hold in the rest of the breath.
- Place food or liquid into the oral cavity (the patient should still be holding the breath).
- Instruct the patient to swallow while holding the breath during the swallow.
- Tell the patient to cough immediately after the swallow.
- Instruct the patient to swallow again (Swigert, 1996).

Note to the Clinician
- Use clinical judgement when deciding to implement this exercise/strategy into the patient's therapy program.
- Make sure that the patient is not at risk for aspiration before implementing this strategy.

Potential Benefits of This Exercise/Strategy
- Increased laryngeal closure
- Decreased risk for aspiration

Protocol for Supraglottic Swallow Exercise/Strategy: *Explanation and Instruction to the Patient*

	Explanation in English	**Explicación en Español**
Clinician	This Supraglottic Swallow Exercise/Strategy helps to close the airway when you swallow. This exercise/strategy may assure that food or liquid does not go into your lungs.	Esta Ejercicio/Estrategia de Trago Supraglottic le ayuda a cerrar la vía aérea. Este ejercicio/estrategia puede asegurarle que la comida o los líquidos no entren a los pulmones.
	Instruction in English	**Instrucción en Español**
Clinician	1. Please take a deep breath and then exhale a little bit of air out. 2. Please hold in the rest of the air and don't let go of it. 3. Please put some food in your mouth. 4. Please continue holding your breath while you swallow your food. 5. Please cough [once the patient finishes swallowing the food]. 6. Please swallow again.	1. Por favor respire profundamente y luego exhale un poco del aire. 2. Por favor detenga el resto del aire y no lo deje ir. 3. Por favor póngase comida en su boca. 4. Por favor continué deteniendo su respiración mientras que traga su comida. 5. Por favor tosa [ya cuando el paciente termine de tragar la comida]. 6. Por favor trague otra vez.

Treatment for Pharyngeal Phase Dysphagia
Increasing Laryngeal Closure
Protocol 5.25 (English/Spanish)

Chin Down Exercise/Strategy

The *Chin Down Exercise/Strategy* is a procedure used to increase laryngeal closure (Bulow, Olsson, & Ekberg 2001; Rasley, Logemann, Kahrilas, Rademaker, Pauloski, & Dodds, 1993; Singh, Brockbank, Frost, & Tyler, 1995; Welch, Logemann, Rademaker, & Kahrilas, 1993).

General Procedures
- Instruct the patient to move the head down and move the chin down toward the chest when food or liquid is consumed.
- Implement this strategy every time the patient puts food or liquid into the mouth.

Note to the Clinician
- Make sure that the patient is sitting up at a 90-degree angle.
- Also make sure that the patient is tucking the chin down and not leaning the head forward (Swigert, 2000).

Potential Benefits of This Exercise/Strategy
- Increased laryngeal closure
- Reduced risk for aspiration

Protocol for Chin Down Exercise/Strategy: *Explanation and Instruction to the Patient*		
	Explanation in English	**Explicación en Español**
Clinician	This Chin Down Exercise/Strategy helps to close the airway when you swallow. This strategy may ensure that food or liquid does not go into your lungs.	Este Ejercicio/Estrategia de Barbilla Hacia Abajo le ayuda a cerrar la vía aérea. Esta estrategia puede asegurarle que la comida o los líquidos no entren a los pulmones.
	Instruction in English	**Instrucción en Español**
Clinician	1. Please sit up as straight as possible. 2. Please put some food in your mouth. 3. Please move your head and chin down toward your chest and swallow. 4. Please do this exercise/strategy every time you put food or liquid into your mouth.	1. Por favor siéntese derecho todo lo que sea posible. 2. Por favor póngase comida en su boca. 3. Por favor mueva su cabeza y su barbilla hacia abajo a su pecho y trague. 4. Por favor use este ejercicio/ estrategia cada vez que se ponga comida o líquido en su boca.

Treatment for Pharyngeal Phase Dysphagia
Increasing Laryngeal Closure
Protocol 5.26 (English/Spanish)

Head Turn Exercise/Strategy

The *Head Turn Strategy* is a set of procedures used to increase laryngeal closure (Logemann, Kahrilas, Kobara, & Vakil 1989; Logemann & Kahrilas, 1990; Rasley, Logemann, Kahrilas, Rademaker, Pauloski, & Dodds, 1993; Silbergleit, Warring, Sullivan, & Maynard, 1991).

General Procedures
- Instruct the patient to turn the head all the way to the right/left side (whichever side is more affected).
- Present food and ask the patient to swallow.
- Implement this strategy during the patient's therapeutic feedings.

Potential Benefits of This Exercise/Strategy
- Increased laryngeal closure
- Decreased risk of aspiration

Protocol for Head Turn Exercise/Strategy: *Explanation and Instruction to the Patient*		
	Explanation in English	**Explicación en Español**
Clinician	This Head Turn Exercise/Strategy helps to close the airway when you swallow. This exercise/strategy may ensure that food or liquid does not go into your lungs.	Este Ejercicio/Estrategia de Voltear la Cabeza le ayuda a cerrar la vía aérea Este ejercicio/estrategia puede asegurarle que la comida o los líquidos no entren a los pulmones.
	Instruction in English	**Instrucción en Español**
Clinician	1. Please sit up straight in your chair. 2. Please turn your head all the way to the left/right side. 3. Please swallow the food that I give you with your head turned completely to the right or left side. 4. Please continue doing this exercise/strategy throughout your meals.	1. Por favor siéntese derecho en su silla. 2. Por favor volteye su cabeza todo lo que se pueda al lado izquierdo/derecho. 3. Por favor trague la comida que le doy con su cabeza volteada al lado derecho o al lado izquierdo. 4. Por favor continué este ejercicio/estrategia durante sus comidas.

Treatment for Pharyngeal Phase Dysphagia
Increasing Laryngeal Closure
Protocol 5.27 (English/Spanish)

Head Turn with Chin Down Exercise/Strategy

The *Head Turn with Chin Down Strategy* is a set of procedures used to increase laryngeal closure (Welch, Logemann, Rademaker, & Kahrilas, 1993; Logemann, 1998).

General Procedures
- Instruct the patient to turn the head all the way to the right/left side (whichever side is more affected).
- Tell the patient to tuck the turned head down toward the chest.
- Present food to the patient.
- The patient uses this strategy during mealtimes.

Potential Benefits of This Exercise/Strategy
- Increased laryngeal closure
- Decreased risk for aspiration

Protocol for Head Turn with Chin Down Exercise/Strategy: *Explanation and Instruction to the Patient*		
	Explanation in English	**Explicación en Español**
Clinician	This Head Turn with Chin Down Exercise/Strategy helps to close the airway when you swallow. This exercise/strategy may ensure that food or liquid does not go into your lungs.	Este Ejercicio/Estrategia de Cabeza Volteada con la Barbilla Hacia Abajo le ayuda a cerrar la vía aérea. Este ejercicio/estrategia puede asegurarle que la comida o los líquidos no entren a los pulmones.
	Instruction in English	**Instrucción en Español**
Clinician	1. Please sit up straight in your chair. 2. Please turn your head all the way to the left/right side. 3. Please put your chin down toward your chest. 4. Please swallow the food that I give you with your head turned completely to the right or left side and your chin down toward your chest. 5. Please continue doing this exercise/strategy during meals.	1. Por favor siéntese derecho en su silla. 2. Por favor volteye su cabeza todo lo que pueda al lado izquierdo/derecho. 3. Por favor ponga la barbilla hacia abajo a su pecho. 4. Por favor trague la comida que le di con su cabeza volteada completamente al lado derecho o izquierdo y la barbilla hacia su pecho. 5. Por favor continué haciendo este ejercicio/estrategia durante sus comidas.

Treatment for Pharyngeal Phase Dysphagia Increasing Laryngeal Elevation

Overview

Patients with pharyngeal phase dysphagia exhibit decreased laryngeal elevation. As a result, the these patients may have poor cricopharyngeal opening with residue in the pyriform sinuses. The patient is at increased risk for aspiration when there is residue in the pyriform sinuses (Logemann, 1998; Swigert, 2000).

This section presents a compensatory swallow therapy exercise and some rehabilitative swallow therapy exercises/strategies that can be used to increase laryngeal elevation.

Compensatory Swallow Therapy Exercise

The following compensatory swallow therapy exercise is described next:

- Falsetto/Pitch Exercises

Rehabilitative Swallow Therapy Exercises/Strategies

The following rehabilitative therapy exercises/strategies also are described:

- Mendelsohn Maneuver Exercise/Strategy
- Super–Supraglottic Strategy
- Supraglottic Strategy

Treatment for Pharyngeal Phase Dysphagia
Increasing Laryngeal Elevation
Protocol 5.28 (English/Spanish)

Falsetto/Pitch Exercise

The *Falsetto/Pitch Exercise* is a set of procedures used to increase laryngeal elevation (Logemann, 1998; Swigert, 2000).

General Procedures

- Instruct the patient to say /i/ with a normal voice and then to gradually say /i/ at a higher pitch. Recognize when the patient reaches the falsetto pitch.
- Tell the patient to hold the production out, once the falsetto pitch has been identified by the clinician.
- Instruct the patient to hold the falsetto production of /i/ for 3 seconds.
- Repeat this exercise three times or as tolerated by the patient.

Potential Benefits of This Exercise

- Increased laryngeal elevation
- Increased airway closure
- Decreased risk for aspiration

Protocol for Falsetto/Pitch Exercise: *Explanation and Instruction to the Patient*		
	Explanation in English	**Explicación en Español**
Clinician	This Falsetto/Pitch Exercise helps to strengthen the muscles in your throat. This exercise may help to reduce the risk of food or liquid going into your airway.	Este Ejercicio de Nivel Falsete le ayuda a aumentar la fuerza de los músculos en su garganta. Este ejercicio puede ayudararle a reducir el riesgo de que la comida o el líquido entren a la vía respiratoria.
	Instruction in English	**Instrucción en Español**
Clinician	1. Please say /i/ with your normal voice. 2. Please sing /i/ and gradually make your voice higher [the clinician sings to show the patient how to do this]. 3. I will tell you to hold out the highest sound you make for 3 seconds. 4. Please repeat this exercise five times.	1. Por favor diga /i/ con voz normal. 2. Por favor cante /i/ y gradualmente haga su voz que se suba más alto [el clínico canta para enseñarle al paciente como hacer esto] 3. Le voy a decir que detenga el sonido mas alto que produce por 3 segundos. 4. Por favor repita este ejercicio cinco veces.

Treatment for Pharyngeal Phase Dysphagia
Increasing Laryngeal Elevation
Protocol 5.29 (English/Spanish)

Mendelsohn Maneuver Exercise/Strategy

The *Mendelsohn Maneuver Exercise/Strategy* is a set of procedures used to increase laryngeal elevation (Bartolome & Neuman, 1993; Bryant, 1991; Ding, Larson, Logemann, & Rademaker, 2002; Logemann, Kahrilas, & Gibbons, 1992).

General Procedures
- Instruct the patient to put a hand on the larynx (do not have the patient hold the larynx).
- Tell the patient to swallow (if using the Mendelsohn maneuver as a strategy, the clinician should present food or liquids).
- Show the patient when the larynx elevates.
- Instruct the patient to swallow and then having the patient identify the highest point when the larynx is elevated.
- Repeat this exercise/strategy five times.
- Instruct the patient to put the hand on the larynx and swallow.
- Have the patient identify the highest point of the swallow and squeeze the muscles in the back of the tongue as hard and as long as possible without the larynx coming back down.
- Repeat this exercise/strategy 10 times.

Note to the Clinician
- This initially is done as an exercise and then is implemented as a compensatory strategy while the patient is eating.

Potential Benefits of This Exercise/Strategy
- Increased laryngeal elevation
- Decreased risk for aspiration

Protocol for Mendelsohn Maneuver Exercise/Strategy: *Explanation and Instruction to the Patient*		
	Explanation in English	**Explicación en Español**
Clinician	This Mendelsohn Maneuver Exercise/ Strategy helps to increase laryngeal elevation. This exercise/strategy may prevent food or liquids from falling into your lungs.	Este Ejercicio/Estrategia de Maniobra Mendelsohn le ayuda a aumentar la elevación de la laringe. Esta ejercicio/ estrategia puede ayudarle a evitar que la comida o los líquidos entren a sus pulmones.
	Instruction in English	**Instrucción en Español**
Clinician	1. Please put your hand on your throat. 2. Please put some food in your mouth [if the Mendelsohn maneuver is being used as a compensatory strategy]. 3. Please swallow and feel your larynx go up. 4. Please show me with your hand where the larynx goes up at the highest point. 5. Please swallow. When your larynx reaches the highest point, please squeeze the back muscles of your tongue for as long and as hard as you can without letting your larynx go down. 6. Please repeat this exercise/strategy five times.	1. Por favor ponga su mano en su garganta. 2. Por favor póngase comida en su boca. [si la Maniobra Mendelsohn se esta usando como estrategia compensatoria]. 3. Por favor trague y sienta como su laringe sube para arriba. 4. Por favor enséñeme con su mano donde la laringe sube al punto mas alto. 5. Por favor trague. Cuando su laringe llegue al punto, mas alto por favor aplane los músculos de atrás de su lengua lo mas fuerte y largo que pueda sin dejar ir la laringe para abajo. 6. Por favor repita este ejercicio/ estrategia cinco veces.

Treatment for Pharyngeal Phase Dysphagia
Increasing Laryngeal Elevation
Protocol 5.30 (English/Spanish)

Super–Supraglottic Swallow Exercise/Strategy

The *Super–Supraglottic Swallow Exercise/Strategy* is a set of procedures used to increase laryngeal elevation (Donzelli & Brady, 2004; Kahrilas, Logemann, & Gibbons, 1992; Logemann, 1998; Martin, Logemann, Shaker, & Dodds, 1993; Swigert, 2000).

General Procedures

- Implement this exercise/strategy to increase tongue base control with patients who have had a supraglottic laryngectomy (Logemann, 1998).
- Have the patient do this exercise without presentation of food.
- Introduce food while incorporating this strategy.
- Instruct the patient to take a deep breath and then exhale out a small amount of air.
- Tell the patient to hold in the breath as tightly as possible.
- Place food or liquid into the oral cavity (the patient should still be holding the breath).
- Instruct the patient to continue holding the breath while squeezing as hard as possible during the swallow.
- Tell the patient to cough and then swallow again (Swigert, 2000).

Note to the Clinician

- This exercise can be done as a compensatory strategy with the patient's recommended diet or during treatment.
- Use clinical judgement when deciding to implement this strategy into the patient's therapy program.
- Make sure that the patient is not at risk for aspiration before implementing this strategy.

Potential Benefits of This Exercise/Strategy

- Increased laryngeal elevation
- Increased laryngeal closure
- Decreased risk for aspiration

Protocol for Super–Supraglottic Swallow Exercise/Strategy: *Explanation and Instruction to the Patient*

	Explanation in English	Explicación en Español
Clinician	This Super–Supraglottic Swallow Exercise/Strategy helps to strengthen your muscles in your throat. This exercise/strategy may prevent food or liquids from falling into your lungs.	Este ejercicio/estrategia de Trago Súper–Supraglottic ayuda a aumentar la fuerza de los músculos en la garganta. Este ejercicio/estrategia puede ayudarle a evitar que la comida o los líquidos entren a sus pulmones.
	Instruction in English	**Instrucción en Español**
Clinician	1. Please take a deep breath in and then exhale a little bit of air out. 2. Please hold in the rest of the air and don't let go of it. 3. I will put some food in your mouth. 4. Please continue holding your breath and squeeze while you are swallowing your food. 5. Please cough [once the patient finishes swallowing the food]. 6. Please swallow again.	1. Por favor inspire y luego deje salir un poco de aire. 2. Por favor detenga el resto del aire y no lo deje salir. 3. Voy a ponerle comida en su boca. 4. Por favor continué deteniendo su respiración y apriete hacia abajo mientras que traga su comida. 5. Por favor tosa [ya cuando el paciente termine de tragar su comida]. 6. Por favor trague otra vez.

Treatment for Pharyngeal Phase Dysphagia
Increasing Laryngeal Elevation
Protocol 5.31 (English/Spanish)

Supraglottic Swallow Exercise/Strategy

The *Supraglottic Swallow Exercise/Strategy* is a set of procedures used to increase laryngeal elevation (Kahrilas, Logemann, & Gibbons, 1992; Singh, Brockbank, Frost, & Tyler, 1995; Swigert, 2000).

General Procedures
- Utilize this exercise without presentation of food and then introduce food while incorporating this strategy.
- Tell the patient to take a deep breath and then exhale a little bit of air out.
- Instruct the patient to hold in the rest of the breath.
- Place food or liquid into the oral cavity (the patient should still be holding in the breath).
- Instruct the patient to swallow while continuing to hold the breath during the swallow.
- Tell the patient to cough immediately after the swallow.
- Instruct the patient to swallow again (Swigert, 2000).

Note to the Clinician
- Use clinical judgement when deciding to implement this strategy into the patient's therapy program.
- Make sure that the patient is not at risk for aspiration before implementing this strategy.

Potential Benefits of This Exercise/Strategy
- Increased laryngeal elevation
- Increased laryngeal closure
- Decreased risk for aspiration

Protocol for Supraglottic Swallow Exercise/Strategy: *Explanation and Instruction to the Patient*		
	Explanation in English	**Explicación en Español**
Clinician	This Supraglottic Swallow Exercise/ Strategy helps to strengthen the muscles in your throat. This exercise/strategy may prevent food or liquids from falling into your lungs.	Esta ejercicio/estrategia le ayuda a aumentar la fuerza de los músculos en la garganta. Este ejercicio/estrategia puede ayudarle a evitar que la comida o los líquidos entren a sus pulmones.
	Instruction in English	**Instrucción en Español**
Clinician	1. Please take a deep breath in and then exhale a little bit of air out. 2. Please hold in the rest of the air and don't let go of it. 3. Please put some food in your mouth. 4. Please continue holding your breath while you swallow your food. 5. Please cough [once the patient finishes swallowing the food]. 6. Please swallow again.	1. Por favor inspire profundamente y luego exhale poco del aire. 2. Por favor detenga el resto del aire y no lo deje ir. 3. Por favor póngase comida en su boca. 4. Por favor continué deteniendo su respiración mientras que traga su comida. 5. Por favor tosa [ya cuando el paciente termine de tragar su comida]. 6. Por favor trague otra vez.

Esophageal Phase Dysphagia

Overview of the Esophageal Phase of Swallowing and Associated Disorders

Disorders affecting the esophageal phase of the swallow typically are managed with medication and surgery. Esophageal phase dysphagia may be diagnosed by the modified barium video fluoroscopic swallow study completed by the radiologist and the speech-language pathologist. The speech-language pathologist should refer patients who exhibit esophageal phase symptoms to a physician or gastroenterologist.

This section presents (a) components of the esophageal phase, (b) signs and symptoms associated with the esophageal phase, (c) disorders associated with the esophageal phase, and (d) general management recommendations.

Components of the Esophageal Phase

The esophageal phase of the swallow consists of the following components:

- The upper esophageal sphincter (UES) relaxes to allow the bolus to enter the esophagus.
- The peristaltic wave moves the bolus through the esophagus.
- The bolus reaches the bottom of the esophagus at the lower esophageal sphincter (LES), where it passes into the stomach.

Signs and Symptoms Associated with the Esophageal Phase Dysphagia

Signs and symptoms associated with the esophageal phase include the following:

- Gastroesophageal reflux
- Burning sensation in the throat
- Feeling of pressure in the throat
- Coughing during the swallow
- Coughing after the swallow
- Choking during the swallow
- Choking after the swallow
- Aspiration

Disorders Associated with the Esophageal Phase

Disorders associated with the esophageal phase include the following:

- Achalasia of the lower esophageal sphincter (LES)
- Gastroesophageal reflex disease (GERD)
- Tracheoesophageal fistula (T-E fistula)
- Zenker's diverticulum

- Esophageal stenosis
- Esophageal tumor
- Esophageal ring
- Esophageal web
- Esophageal spasm

General Management Recommendations

Disorders of the esophagus normally are not treated by the speech-language pathologist. However, the speech-language pathologist can give the patient some general recommendations to reduce symptoms due to gastroesophageal reflux (refer to Therapy Resource 5.1 [English/Spanish]).

Esophageal Phase Dysphagia
Treatment Resource 5.1 (English/Spanish)

Recommendations to Prevent Gastroesophageal Reflux

• Avoid the following foods and liquids:
  ➢ Chocolate
  ➢ Peppermint
  ➢ Fatty foods
  ➢ Coffee
  ➢ Alcoholic beverages
  ➢ Pepper
  ➢ Citrus fruits
  ➢ Citrus juices
  ➢ Tomato products
  ➢ Chile or spices
  ➢ Acidic or sour foods
	• Evite las siguientes comidas y líquidos:
	  ➢ Chocolate
	  ➢ Hierba-buena
	  ➢ Comidas grasosas
	  ➢ Café
	  ➢ Bebidas alcohólicas
	  ➢ Pimienta
	  ➢ Frutas agrias
	  ➢ Jugos agrios
	  ➢ Productos de tomate
	  ➢ Chile y especias
	  ➢ Comidas ácidas o agrias

• Decrease the portions of food at mealtimes.	• Disminuye las porciones de comida cuando come.
• Eat meals 2 to 3 hours before going to bed.	• Coma sus comidas 2 a 3 horas antes de acostarse.
• Lose weight if you are overweight.	• Pierda peso si esta demasiado pesado.
• Decrease or stop smoking.	• Disminuye o deje de fumar.
• Elevate the head of the bed on 6-inch blocks.	• Levante la cabeza de la cama sobre bloques de 6 pulgadas.
• Sleep on a specially designed wedge (which can be purchased in a pharmacy).	• Duerma en una cuna especial de esponja (que se puede comprar en la farmacia).
• Stay in an upright position for 30 minutes after eating.	• Quédese en una posición derecha por 30 minutos después de que coma.
• Avoid wearing tight-fitting clothes.	• Evite ropa que le queda apretada.

Section 6

Inservice Resources on Staff Education

The speech-language pathologist must educate all staff members about the management of patients with swallowing disorders. It is important to instruct the staff on the nature of the swallowing disorders affecting a patient, specific safe feeding techniques, and compensatory strategies. Staff education is critical because the speech-language pathologist cannot provide services to the patient during all mealtimes. The health care staff is there for the patient at every meal. Therefore, the staff needs to understand the recommendations the speech-language pathologist has made for the patient. The risks of aspiration and choking are decreased when the staff is well trained. The staff training includes physicians as well, because they are ultimately responsible to manage dysphagia in their patients.

Inservice outlines and posttests for eight different areas of concern in the treatment of dysphagia are presented in this section. Each inservice outline and posttest can be modified and printed out for use by the speech-language pathologist in the work setting. The inservice topics include the following:

- Working with Multidisciplinary Teams
- Safety and Precautions of Feeding
- Feeding the Disoriented Patient
- Feeding Techniques and Safe Swallowing
- Terminology and Documentation for the Restorative Feeding Program.
- What You Should Know About Patients on Thick Liquids
- Swallowing After Trauma and CVA
- Physician Education on the Role of the Speech-Language Pathologist and Swallowing

Staff Education

Working with a Dysphagia Multidisciplinary Team

This inservice session may be conducted for nurses, certified nursing assistants, and restorative nursing assistants. The cooperation among these specialists will provide better outcomes for the patient with dysphagia. The purpose of this inservice feature is to outline the roles that each team member plays in safely managing the patient with dysphagia. The staff should know the referral process for patients with swallowing difficulties.

This inservice outline may be reproduced and can be turned in to the director of staff development for facility records. There is a posttest that may be reproduced and administered to the inservice participants to evaluate the effects of the program. This may become a record of attendance in the participant's file or may be used to fulfill continuing education requirements for recertification or renewal of state licenses.

Staff Education
Inservice Resource 6.1

Working with a Dysphagia Multidisciplinary Team

Target Staff: Nurses, CNAs, and RNAs; working with a treatment team

Purpose: To train members of the target staff on their role as part of the dysphagia team and to emphasize how their efforts will improve oral intake for the patients

Objectives: By the end of the inservice, the staff will:

- Identify members on the dysphagia management team
- Understand the roles of the dysphagia management team
- Identify symptoms for patient referral

The Dysphagia Management Team

The dysphagia management team typically includes a variety of specialists.

The Director of Nurses

The director of nurses is responsible for the following:

- overseeing the dysphagia management team
- supervising the dysphagia management team

The Director of Education/Staff Development

The director of education/staff development is responsible for the following:

- implementing in-services to educate the staff
- providing continuing education for the staff

The Charge Nurse

The charge nurse is responsible for the following:

- providing overall patient care
- supervising the certified nursing assistants who care for the patients
- reporting weight losses and weight gains to the physician and the registered dietitian
- reporting change of conditions in swallowing or feeding to the speech-language pathologist or the occupational therapist when reported by the certified nursing assistants or observed by the nurse

The Certified Nursing Assistant (CNA)

The certified nursing assistant is responsible for the following:

- providing daily care for the patients who are assigned to that nursing assistant (e.g., assistance with showers, dressing)
- reporting change in condition on patients' swallowing or feeding to the charge nurse, speech-language pathologist, or occupational therapist
- reporting the patients' weight data to the charge nurse

The Restorative Nursing Assistant (RNA)

The restorative nursing assistant is responsible for the following:

- monitoring the patient in the restorative dining program
- reporting change in condition in the patient's swallowing or feeding to the charge nurse, speech-language pathologist, or occupational therapist

The Speech-Language Pathologist (SLP)

The speech-language pathologist is responsible for the following:

- screening patients who have difficulty chewing or swallowing their food
- evaluating patients who have difficulty chewing or swallowing their food
- treating patients who have difficulty chewing or swallowing their food

The Occupational Therapist (OT)

The occupational therapist is responsible for the following:

- screening patients who are having difficulty feeding themselves
- evaluating patients who are having difficulty feeding themselves
- treating patients who are having difficulty feeding themselves

The Registered Dietitian

The registered dietitian is responsible for the following:

- making sure the patient is on the right type of diet
- checking the patient's hydration and nutritional status

Symptoms of Dysphagia

The staff should refer patients to the dysphagia team if the patient is:

- refusing to eat food and drink liquids
- spilling food or liquid outside of the mouth

- pocketing food inside the cheek
- refusing to open the mouth to eat or drink
- holding food or liquid inside the mouth for a long time and not swallowing
- coughing when liquids are swallowed
- coughing when food is swallowed
- having congestion after eating food or drinking liquids
- choking on food
- reporting that food feels "stuck in the throat"
- having difficulty taking medications
- having recurring episodes of pneumonia
- losing weight
- drooling
- slurring words during conversation

The Patient Referral

Nursing staff members who suspect swallowing problems in a patient should refer the patient to:

- the charge nurse, who, after receiving a referral from the certified nursing assistants and restorative nursing assistants, will then refer the patient for screening
- the speech-language pathologist, who is responsible for checking the patient's swallowing abilities
- the occupational therapist, who is responsible for checking the ability of the patient to self-feed

Staff Education
Posttest

Working with a Dysphagia Multidisciplinary Team

1. List all of the members of the dysphagia management team:

   _____   _____

   _____   _____

   _____   _____

2. Match the team members with their roles.

   A. Director of nurses   ___ In charge of education of staff

   B. Director of education   ___ In charge of patients in their care

   C. Charge nurse   ___ Oversees the dysphagia team

   D. CNA   ___ In charge of patient's swallowing abilities

   E. RNA   ___ In charge of patient's appropriate diet

   F. SLP   ___ In charge of patient's feeding skills

   G. OT   ___ In charge of patient's restorative dining

   H. Registered dietitian   ___ Responsible for patient's daily care
                                       (e.g., assistance with showers, dressing)

3. List three symptoms to look for to refer a patient to the dysphagia management team:

   _____

   _____

   _____

4. To whom do you refer a patient with swallowing problems? _____

   _____

   _____

5. To whom do you refer a patient with feeding problems? _____

   _____

   _____

Staff Education 1

Safety and Precautions with Feeding

This inservice session may be conducted with all nursing staff. The cooperation of all members of the nursing staff will provide a safer environment and ensure safe feeding precautions for the patient with dysphagia. This inservice features outlines proper positioning of the patient, appropriate environment, and safe and unsafe feeding strategies to manage the patient with dysphagia. The staff should know the do's and don'ts of feeding a patient with dysphagia.

The inservice outline may be reproduced and turned in to the director of staff development for facility records. There is a posttest that may be copied for the inservice participants to complete. This may become a record of attendance in the participant's file or may be used to fulfill continuing education requirements for recertification or state license renewal.

Staff Education 1
Inservice Resource 6.2

Safety and Precautions with Feeding

Target Staff: All nursing staff

Purpose: To train the staff on how to safely feed a patient

Objectives: By the end of the inservice session, the staff will understand:

- The positioning of patients for safe feeding
- Dining environment appropriate for patients
- Feeding techniques that are appropriate and inappropriate to use with patients

Positioning the Patient for Safe Feeding

All patients with dysphagia should be correctly positioned for safe feeding.

- Positioning the patient in **bed** for safe feeding:
  - ➢ Position the patient to an upright 90-degree angle in bed.
  - ➢ Raise the patient's feet in bed so that the knees are slightly flexed to keep the patient from scooting down.
- Positioning the patient in a **chair** for safe feeding:
  - ➢ Position the patient in an upright 90-degree angle in a chair/wheelchair.
  - ➢ Make sure that the patient's feet are on the floor or on the wheelchair foot rests.
- Positioning the patient at the **table** for safe feeding:
  - ➢ Position the patient so the table is at the patient's ribcage or waist level.

Environment for Social Dining

Create an enjoyable social dining experience for the patient:

- The environment should be quiet and pleasant.
- Music should be soft and mellow.
- The patient should be relaxed and not feel rushed at mealtimes.
- Staff conversations should be directed to patients about the meal (staff conversations should not be about personal problems or circumstances).
- The atmosphere should be sociable, as in a restaurant or a dining room at home.

Safety for Feeding

To ensure safe swallowing during mealtimes, the staff should:

- allow the patient plenty of time to eat
- encourage the patient to eat and drink
- inform the patient about what is on the menu for the meal/day
- help the patient open all containers on the tray (if assistance is needed)
- make positive remarks about the patient's food (the way it looks and smells)
- monitor closely the patient who is having difficulty swallowing
- feed the patient slowly, or give verbal cues to self-feeding patients to slow down
- present one teaspoon of food at a time, or give verbal cues to take only one spoon at a time
- check to make sure the food or liquid is not too hot before it is fed to the patient
- place the patient's food in an area where the patient can see and reach the food
- check to see if the patient has dentures or partials on if they need them
- check to see if the patient is wearing corrective lenses at meals if they are needed
- allow the patient enough space to eat in by reducing overcrowding
- offer the patient an alternate choice of food if he or she does not like the food on the menu for that meal
- inform the nurse if the patient is not eating or drinking

Precautions for Feeding

To ensure the patient's safety during swallowing, the nursing staff should observe the following precautions:

- do not rush the patient
- do not use large spoons to feed the patient
- do not put more than one spoon of food in the patient's mouth at one time
- do not walk away after putting the tray of food down in front of the patient (the patient may need tray setup or assistance with the containers on the tray)
- do not make negative comments about how the food looks are smells
- do not take the patient's tray away without asking if the patient is through eating
- do not talk about personal matters during the patient's mealtime
- do not take lightly the fact that the patient refuses to eat or drink

Staff Education 1
Posttest

Safety and Precautions with Feeding

1. Patients should be sitting in bed for meals at a:

   A. 45° angle

   B. 60° angle

   C. 90° angle

2. *True* or *False*: The table should be close to the patient's mouth, so the patient can reach the mouth faster.

3. *True* or *False*: It is all right to discuss your personal problems in the patient's dining area while the patients eat.

4. The atmosphere in the dining room should be:

   A. Quiet.

   B. Pleasant.

   C. Rushed.

   D. Both A and B.

5. List three safety techniques to use while feeding the patient.

   _____

   _____

   _____

6. List three precautions to use while feeding the patient.

   _____

   _____

   _____

Staff Education 2

Feeding the Disoriented Patient

Feeding a disoriented patient may pose unique challenges. This inservice training session may be conducted for all nursing staff. The cooperation of the nursing staff will provide the appropriate environment and ensure safe feeding for the patient with dysphagia who is disoriented. This inservice feature outlines when and how the nursing staff may approach the patient with disorientation, strategies that may be used for safe swallowing, and the importance of reality orientation techniques to use with the patient. The staff should be familiar with the special needs of the patient with disorientation. The staff members should know how to redirect the agitated patient.

The inservice outline may be reproduced and turned in to the director of staff development for facility records. There is a post-test for the inservice participants to complete. This may become a record of attendance in the participant's file or may be used to fulfill continuing education requirements for recertification or state license renewal.

Staff Education 2
Inservice Resource 6.3

Feeding the Disoriented Patient

Target Staff: All nursing staff

Purpose: To train the nursing staff on compensatory strategies to use in feeding the patient with decreased attention, decreased cognition, decreased physical functions, and disorientation to place, person, or time

Objectives: By the end of the inservice session, the staff will understand:

- When and how to safely assist the disoriented patient with dysphagia
- Compensatory strategies that promote safe swallowing
- The importance of reality orientation techniques

When and How to Safely Assist the Disoriented Patient with Dysphagia

To safely assist the disoriented patient, the staff should incorporate the following into their practice:

- Recognize that these patients have special needs and need special approaches.
- Treat the patient in a respectful manner.
- Approach the patient calmly.
- Speak softly and slowly to the patient.
- Remind the patient that it is time to eat.
- Invite the patient to join others for the meal.
- Assist the patient who needs help in setting up his or her meal tray.
- Recognize that the patient often will be hesitant to cooperate during mealtimes.
- Leave the patient alone when he or she is uncooperative, but return after few minutes and offer assistance in getting to the dining room.
- Appreciate that the patient who does not understand what he or she is expected to do tends to be combative.
- Recognize that the patient may not understand that help is being offered.
- Leave the patient alone for a few minutes if the patient is combative, thus allowing the patient time to calm down.
- Approach the patient a few minutes later with a glass of juice or a piece of food from the meal tray, which may remind the patient that it is time to eat.

Strategies to Promote Safe Swallowing

To promote safe swallowing, the following strategies may be useful for the staff:

- Make the patient's environment as pleasant as possible.
- Restrict the amount of disruptions or noises around the patient.
- Train the staff to adopt attitudes and approaches to the patient that are slow and gentle.
- Enforce the seating arrangement at these patients' tables for consistency, as these patients function better with structure and consistency in their daily routines.
- Position the patient comfortably in a chair, near the food, with all items on the tray within reach.
- Place only one plate of food and one glass or cup of liquid at a time in front of the patient to reduce chances of becoming overwhelmed.
- Keep verbal instructions simple and give one command at a time, spoken slowly.
- Allow the patient to get up and walk around while eating or drinking, and inform the speech-language pathologist so that a finger food diet may be considered for this type of patient.
- Allow the patient to self-feed as much as possible, and assist the patient when he or she fatigues or forgets to continue eating.

Use of Reality Orientation Techniques

To improve the patient's reality orientation, the staff should:

- Approach the patient calmly in a soothing voice.
- Call the patient by name (e.g., "Mr. _____" or "Mrs. _____").
- Inform the patient that it is time to eat (i.e., "It is noon and time for you to eat your lunch").
- Inform the patient that you are his or her nursing assistant and that you are going to help get to the dining room (e.g., "I am your assistant today; I will help you go to the dining room for your lunch").
- Tell the patient what the menu being shown is for that meal (e.g., "Today you are having roast beef with gravy, mashed potatoes, mixed vegetables, a roll and butter, apple pie, coffee, and ice tea for lunch").
- Encourage the patient to eat by stating that the food looks or smells good (e.g., "Your food looks and smells yummy").

Staff Education 2
Posttest

Feeding the Disoriented Patient

1. *True* or *False*: The disoriented patient is so confused, it doesn't matter how you speak to him or her.

2. What do you do when disoriented patients do not cooperate with you when you try to assist them to the dining room?

   A. Leave them alone. If they don't eat, they just don't eat.

   B. Leave them alone. Return again and offer to take them to the dining room.

   C. Insist that they go to the dining room; if you can, push them over to the dining room.

3. What do you do when patients get combative and do not want to go to the dining room?

   A. Leave them alone.

   B. Return later.

   C. Try bringing a drink or food with you to remind them it is time to eat.

   D. All of the above.

4. *True* or *False*: The patient's food should be within reach.

5. *True* or *False*: The whole tray of food and liquid should be placed in front of the patient so the patient can eat or drink what he or she wants.

6. *True* or *False*: The daily seating arrangements for these patients at meals should be the same.

7. *True* or *False*: It is okay for the disoriented patient to get up and walk around at meal times.

8. *True* or *False*: Always tell the patient what is on the menu for that meal.

9. *True* or *False*: It doesn't matter whether you address the patient by name because he or she is too confused anyway.

10. *True* or *False*: If the food looks gross to you, tell the patient.

Staff Education 3

Safe Feeding Techniques and Precautions

This inservice session may be conducted for all nursing staff. After completing the session, the nursing staff will be knowledgeable about aspiration and choking precautions. The staff also will be able to assist the patient in learning how to safely swallow. This inservice feature will allow the participants to recognize the importance of oral hygiene for the patient before a meal.

The inservice outline may be reproduced and can be turned in to the director of staff development for facility records. There is a posttest that may be copied for the inservice participants to complete. This may become a record of attendance in the participant's file or may be used to fulfill continuing education requirements for recertification or state license renewal.

Staff Education 3
Inservice Resource 6.4

Safe Feeding Techniques and Precautions

Target Staff: Nursing staff, CNAs, and RNAs

Purpose: To train the staff to understand and use safe swallow techniques with patients who have swallowing difficulties

Objectives: By the end of the inservice, the staff will:

- Take safe swallow precautions
- Use oral hygiene procedures
- Assist the patient in learning how to safely swallow
- Monitor the patient's oral intake

Precautions

To ensure safe swallowing for the patient, the staff should take the following precautions:

Aspiration precautions
- Sit the patient in a 90-degree angle upright position.
- Have the patient sit up for 30 to 45 minutes after the meal.
- Make sure that the patient receives the appropriate diet.

Choking precautions
- Make sure the patient chews food sufficiently and then swallows.
- Instruct the patient to slow down the rate.
- Instruct the patient to eat only one teaspoon of food at a time.

Dining Setting

Arrange the dining setting so that it is:

- Quiet
- Positive
- Pleasant

Oral Hygiene Before Feeding the Patient

Before feeding the patient, the nursing staff should:

- check the patient's mouth before he or she begins to eat to see if it is clean, to reduce the risk of infection

- clean the patient's mouth if it is not clean before the patient begins to eat, to improve the taste of foods eaten and to reduce the risk of infection
- check the patient's mouth at the end of a meal to clean and remove any food that may be in the mouth, to reduce the risk of aspiration and choking

Feeding the Patient

To safely feed the patient, the staff should:

- position the patient in an upright 90-degree angle sitting position in a chair or bed and place pillows around the patient to maintain this position
- move the patient's head slightly forward
- position the patient's knees slightly flexed up in bed to keep the patient from sliding down in bed

In presenting food to the patient, the staff should:

- follow the patient's diet as recommended by the speech-language pathologist
- show and tell the patient everything that is on the tray
- present only one small spoonful at a time
- check to see if the patient has finished all of the food before more food is given
- provide verbal cues to remind the patient to close the lips around the spoon
- provide verbal cues to the patient to chew food
- instruct the patient with verbal cues to start a swallow and then to swallow
- give verbal cues to the patient to use a tongue sweep to clear food from the gums and cheeks
- touch the patient's cheek to remind the patient to clear food from that cheek
- use the index finger to stroke the patient's throat from the Adam's apple upward toward the base of the tongue, to initiate a swallow
- follow specific compensatory strategies recommended by the speech-language pathologist

In presenting liquids to the patient, the staff should:

- present liquids as ordered by the speech-language pathologist
- use a glass, cup, spoon, or straw as recommended by the speech-language pathologist
- use compensatory strategies that are outlined by the speech-language pathologist while the patient is eating or drinking liquids

Additional Instructions for the Staff

- Allow the patient plenty of time to eat.
- Note that the food and liquids should come from the dietary department as ordered by the speech-language pathologist, and the staff should not thin, thicken, or mash foods or liquids on the patient's tray in the dining room or the patient's room.
- Inform the charge nurse if the patient's tray comes with an incorrect diet or liquid consistency so that another tray may be requested from the dietary department.

Staff Education 3
Posttest
Safe Feeding Techniques and Precautions

1. Two precautions to take when working with patients who have swallowing problems are: _____ and _____ .

2. What position should patient be in to eat? _____

   _____

3. List 3 techniques to use when giving the patient food.

   _____

   _____

   _____

4. What type of liquids should a patient be offered? _____

   _____

5. When should the patient's mouth be cleaned? _____

   _____

6. When should you check the patient's mouth?
   A. Before the meal begins
   B. During the meal
   C. After the meal
   D. All of the above

7. *True* or *False*: It is okay to speed up the feeding process for your patient if you need to be at a staff meeting.

8. *True* or *False*: You should not mash, thicken, or thin the patient's food or liquids.

9. *True* or *False*: If the food or liquids for the patient are incorrect, you should let the charge nurse know after you feed the patient.

10. *True* or *False*: Providing good oral care to my patients decreases the risk of infection.

Staff Education 4

Documentation for the Restorative Feeding Program

This inservice session may be conducted for the restorative nursing assistants (RNAs). The cooperation of the RNAs will provide the dysphagia team with more supervised time with the patient at mealtimes. The RNAs will become familiar with the forms used for documentation in this program. This inservice feature will train them on how to complete the forms for the feeding program. The RNAs also will learn where the forms for the program should be kept. This inservice training is easy to follow and conduct.

The inservice outline may be reproduced and can be turned in to the director of staff development for facility records. There is a posttest that may be copied for the inservice participants to complete. This may become a record of attendance in the participant's file or may be used to fulfill continuing education requirements for recertification or state license renewal.

Staff Education 4
Inservice Resource 6.5

Documentation for the Restorative Feeding Program

Target Staff: RNAs

Purpose: To train the RNAs in procedures for documentation used in the restorative feeding program

Objectives: By the end of the inservice session, the staff will:

- Know the forms to be used in the restorative feeding program
- Know how to complete the forms that are used in the restorative feeding program

The Forms Used in the Restorative Dining Program

The forms that may be used in this program include:

- The Restorative Program Initial Assessment Form. This form should be:
  - ➤ completed by the speech-language pathologist or the occupational therapist
  - ➤ filed by the RNA in the restorative feeding program binder until the patient is discharged from the program
  - ➤ filed in the patient's medical record chart on discharge from the restorative feeding program (the RNA may file the form in the current medical record chart, or route it to medical records)
- The Restorative Nursing Assistant Care Plan Form. This form informs the RNA about the plan of care for the patient, regarding the patient's swallowing difficulties. This form should be:
  - ➤ completed by a speech-language pathologist filed by the RNA in the restorative feeding program binder, until the patient is discharged from the program
  - ➤ reviewed carefully by the RNA on a daily basis
  - ➤ filed in the patient's medical file in the patient's medical record chart on discharge from the restorative feeding program (the RNA can file the form in the current medical chart or route it to medical records)
- The Restorative Feeding Program Daily Notes. The form should be divided into the three meals per day (breakfast, lunch, and dinner). This form, completed by the RNA, should:
  - ➤ cover a 1-month period. A space is provided for the appropriate month and year to be written
  - ➤ have the patient's name, room number, bed number, and physician's name (use a separate form for each patient)
  - ➤ include the RNA's initials on a daily basis to provide documentation that care was completed by the assistant for that day
  - ➤ provide goals for the patient that the RNAs should follow
  - ➤ indicate a code for patient response to the program:

R = refused. Write the reason why the patient refused in the RNA progress note. The RNA should document that the charge nurse was informed of the patient's refusal to eat or participate in the program.

O = out of facility. Write where the patient was at the mealtime in the RNA progress note. The RNA should also write that the charge nurse was aware that the patient did not participate in the program because he or she was out of the facility.

W = withheld. Write the reason why the treatment in the restorative dining room was withheld. The RNA also should document that the charge nurse was informed that the treatment in the program was withheld.

➤ provide codes for type of assistance used with the patient:

MX = maximum assistance. This indicates the patient required hands-on assistance with 75% of the meal.

MD = moderate physical assistance. This indicates the patient required hands-on assistance with 50% of the meal.

MI = minimum physical assistance. This indicates the patient required hands-on assistance with 25% of the meal.

VP = verbal prompts only. This indicates the patient required no hands-on assistance, only verbal cues to finish the meal.

Other: A space is provided for other cues that might be used with the patient.

➤ provide a code for patient participation section:

EN = eats neatly. The patient eats neatly, with little or no spillage of food or liquid.

EM = "eats messy." The patient eats messily, with spillage of food or liquid evident.

C = confused. The patient needs to be provided with reality orientation often (e.g., "You are in the dining room to eat lunch").

F = forgets to take the next bite. The patient requires verbal cues to take the next bite; otherwise, the patient does not attend to the meal.

D = distractable. The patient is easily distracted and requires verbal cues to stay focused on the task of eating or drinking.

- The restorative nursing assistant should document the following information on the form:
  ➤ percentage of food and liquid consumed during meals
  ➤ type of assistance provided during meals
  ➤ patient participation during mealtimes
- Each sheet of the form should have a section for adaptive devices and special assistance, where the restorative nursing assistant can list any special plates, utensils, or cups that the patient uses during meal times.
- Each sheet should be filed in the patient's medical chart at the end of the month or at discharge or should be routed to the medical records division.

Staff Education 4
Posttest

Documentation for the Restorative Feeding Program

A blank Restorative Feeding Program Daily Notes Form is provided. Complete the form based on the following information:

- The patient's name is George Lowe.
- The room number is 13.
- The bed number is 2.
- The physician is Dr. Loya.
- The date is December 8, 2006.
- The patient consumed 25% of his lunch meal.
- The patient required maximal assistance with verbal prompts.
- The patient was very messy when he ate.
- The patient forgot to take the next bite.
- The RNA needs to use his or her own initial and signature.
- The goals are as follows:
  - ➤ The patient must be verbally reminded: "Swallow."
  - ➤ The patient must use a chin tuck on every swallow.
  - ➤ The patient requires the RNA to lightly touch the back of the patient's head as a reminder to use the chin tuck on the swallow.

Staff Education 4
Recording Protocol 6.1

Restorative Feeding Program Initial Assessment

Physician's Orders: _____ Date: _____

Diagnosis: _____ Onset Date: _____

Precautions: Aspiration: ☐ Yes ☐ No   Choking: ☐ Yes ☐ No

Prior Level of Function: _____

_____

Glasses:	☐ Yes ☐ No	
Hearing Aid:	☐ Yes ☐ No	
Partials:	☐ Yes ☐ No ☐ Upper ☐ Lower	
Dentures:	☐ Yes ☐ No ☐ Upper ☐ Lower	

Adaptive Equipment: _____

Handedness: ☐ Right ☐ Left

Right/Left Reason for Referral: _____

Current Feeding Ability: **Oral Motor Screen:**

	Able	Unable		Yes	No
Chew	☐	☐	Drooling	☐	☐
Eat with spoon	☐	☐	Mouth closure	☐	☐
Eat with fork	☐	☐	Coughing	☐	☐
Drink from a cup	☐	☐	Choking	☐	☐
Cut with a knife	☐	☐	Delayed swallow	☐	☐
Drink from a straw	☐	☐	Tongue mobility	☐	☐
Open containers	☐	☐	Gurgly "wet" voice	☐	☐

I. Recommendations: Patient to be given restorative feeding program effective date:

_____

_____

II. Goals: _____

Patient: _____ Room #: _____ Patient #: _____

Therapist _____ Date: _____

Staff Education 4
Recording Protocol 6.2

RNA Care Plan

Initial & Date	Concern or Problem	Goal	Approaches
	• chewing skills • prolonged chewing • coughing on regular liquid • throat clearing on regular liquids • oral retention of bolus • food spilling from the mouth __ left __ right • liquid spilling from mouth __ left __ right • food pocketing __ left __ right • liquid pocketing __ left __ right • food sticking to roof of mouth • unable to remove food utensil (weak lip seal) • not opening mouth to eat or drink • significant weight loss	Patient will safely consume oral diet free of: • choking • aspiration • weight loss • pneumonia • increased congestion • malnutrition • dehydration • increased confusion • (Review × ____ wk)	• RNA program for restorative dining ____ × a day for: ➤ Breakfast ➤ Lunch ➤ Dinner • Refer to patient assessment by: ➤ SLP ➤ OT • Refer to patient's specific program in chart • D/C from RNA program

Name: _____ Medical Record #: _____

Physician: _____ Room #: _____

Staff Education 4
Recording Protocol 6.3

Restorative Feeding Program Daily Notes

CODE

R = refused
O = out of facility

TYPE OF ASSISTANCE

MX = maximum—Fed/75% hands-on assistance
MD = moderate physical assistance
MI = minimum physical assistance
VP = verbal prompts only
Other (specify): _____

PATIENT PARTICIPATION

EN = eats neatly
EM = "eats messy"
C = confused
F = forgets to take next bite
D = distractable
Other (specify): _____

Month/Year: _____

	1	2	3	4	5	6	7	8	9	10	11	12	13	14	15	16	17	18	19	20	21	22	23	24	25	26	27	28	29	30	31
BREAKFAST																															
0% Consumed																															
0% Self Feed																															
0% Assisted																															
Type of Assistance																															
Pt's Participation																															
INITIALS																															
LUNCH																															
0% Consumed																															
0% Self Feed																															
0% Assisted																															
Type of Assistance																															
Pt's Participation																															
INITIALS																															
DINNER																															
0% Consumed																															
0% Self Feed																															
0% Assisted																															
Type of Assistance																															
Pt's Participation																															
INITIALS																															

Adaptive Devices: Special Assistance: _____

INT	SIGNATURE	INT	SIGNATURE	INT	SIGNATURE
Initial and sign once, each page					

RESTORATIVE FEEDING PROGRAM GOALS: _____

Patient's Name: _____ Room #: _____ Bed #: _____ Physician: _____

Staff Education 5

What Dietary Staff Should Know About Patients on Thick Liquids

This inservice session may be conducted with the dietary staff. The dietary staff is responsible for providing the patient with the appropriate food and liquid consistencies. The purpose of this inservice feature is to inform members of the dietary staff about the following: (1) why patients are placed on special food and liquid consistencies, (2) consequences of not delivering the appropriate food and liquid consistencies, and (3) precautions the dietary staff must consider for patients with special diets.

The inservice outline may be reproduced and can be turned in to the director of staff development for facility records. There is a post-test that may be copied for the participants in the inservice session to complete. This may become a record of attendance in the participant's file or may be used to fulfill continuing education requirements for recertification or state license renewal.

Staff Education 5
Inservice Resource 6.6

What Dietary Staff Should Know About Patients on Thick Liquids

Target Staff: Dietary staff

Purpose: To train the members of the dietary staff about the importance of appropriate food and liquid consistencies and how their job influences patient care and safety

Objective: By the end of the inservice session, the staff will understand:

- Why patients are placed on special food and liquid consistencies
- What the consequences are of not delivering the appropriate food and liquid consistencies
- What patients on thick liquids can and cannot have

Why Patients Are Placed on Special Diets

The speech-language pathologist evaluates patients with swallowing difficulties. Patients need special diets because of the specified difficulties they may have:

- Problems in the oral or mouth area may include:
  - difficulty chewing the food
  - spillage of food or liquid out of the mouth.
  - difficulty chewing and putting the food together before swallowing (because of no teeth or dentures or loose fitting dentures)
  - difficulty because of a toothache
  - difficulty because of sores in the mouth
- Management of problems in the oral or mouth area may require:
  - liquid diet
  - pureed diet
  - fine-chopped diet (dental soft)
  - mechanical soft diet
- Reasons for dietary changes may include:
  - weight loss
  - malnutrition
  - dehydration
  - confusion
  - choking
  - aspiration
- Problems in the throat area may include:
  - sensation of food getting stuck in the throat area
  - coughing or throat clearing after the swallow
  - choking on food or liquids
  - wet or gurgly voice after the swallow

- Management of problems in the throat area may require:
  - ➢ liquid diet
  - ➢ pureed diet
  - ➢ fine-chopped (dental soft) diet
  - ➢ mechanical soft diet
  - ➢ thickened liquids
- Reasons for dietary change may include:
  - ➢ choking
  - ➢ aspiration
  - ➢ weight loss
  - ➢ malnutrition
  - ➢ dehydration
  - ➢ confusion

Patients on Thick Liquids

Thickened liquids are recommended when the patient is having difficulty swallowing regular liquids. The patient who needs thick liquids could develop pneumonia and die if the liquids are not thickened as recommended by the speech-language pathologist. The patient's throat muscles are weak and cannot manage regular liquids. The patient has to have a doctor's order to receive thick liquids. This order is as important as the one for medicine. The following forms of liquids must be available:

- regular liquids
- nectar: thickened to manufacturers' specifications
- honey-thick liquids: thickened to manufacturers' specifications
- pudding-thick liquids: thickened to manufacturers' specifications

Patients on thick liquids

- Patients on thick liquids may have:
  - ➢ pudding
  - ➢ yogurt
  - ➢ whipped Jell-O
  - ➢ canned fruit that has been strained
- Patients on thick liquids may **not** have:
  - ➢ ice cream
  - ➢ sherbet
  - ➢ raw or canned fruit that contains a lot of juice
  - ➢ cold cereal (unless thickened milk is used)
  - ➢ unthickened soups, stews, and gravies

Staff Education 5
Posttest

What Dietary Staff Should Know About Patients on Thick Liquids

1. Name three problems a patient with swallowing difficulty in the mouth may have.

   _____

   _____

   _____

2. *True* or *False*: If the patient with chewing and swallowing problems in the mouth area does not get soft food, he or she could lose weight, become more confused, or choke.

3. The complaint of the patient who has trouble swallowing in the throat area is called

   _____

4. *True* or *False*: If the patient with chewing and swallowing problems in the mouth area does not get soft food, he or she could choke and die.

5. What are the four consistencies of liquids?

   _____   _____

   _____   _____

6. *True* or *False*: The patient who needs thick liquids could develop pneumonia and die if his or her liquids are not thickened as recommended by the speech-language pathologist.

7. *True* or *False*: The patient on thick liquids cannot have whipped Jell-O, pudding, and yogurt.

8. *True* or *False*: The patient on thick liquids can have ice cream and sherbet.

9. *True* or *False*: Thick liquids are a doctor's order for the patient, just like the patient's medicines are a doctor's order.

10. *True* or *False*: A patient on thick liquids can have regular liquids every now and then without being in any kind of danger.

Staff Education 6

Swallowing After Trauma and CVA

This inservice session may be conducted with all members of the nursing staff. It is important for the nursing staff to understand the swallowing problems that a patient who has had a cerebrovascular accident (CVA) or head trauma may experience. The purpose of this inservice feature is to inform the nursing staff about the swallowing difficulties a patient with head trauma or CVA may exhibit and the strategies that may be used to promote safe swallowing with these patients.

The inservice outline may be reproduced and can be turned in to the director of staff development for facility records. There is a posttest that may be copied for the inservice participants to complete. This may become a record of attendance in the participant's file or may be used to fulfill continuing education requirements for recertification or state license renewal.

Staff Education 6
Inservice Resource 6.7

Swallowing After Trauma and CVA

Target Staff: All nursing staff

Purpose: To educate the staff on swallowing difficulties of patients with CVA and head trauma and to train them on compensatory strategies for safe swallowing for these patients.

Objectives: By the end of the inservice session, the staff will:

- Identify the swallowing difficulties of the patient who has had a CVA or tramatic head injury
- Understand compensatory strategies to promote safe swallowing

Swallowing Difficulties After a CVA

After a CVA, the patient may have one or more of the following difficulties:

- poor head and body positioning, causing the patient to lean to the right or the left
- neglect on the affected side, which may cause difficulty seeing food or other objects on the affected side
- visual, perceptual, and spatial problems, which may cause self-feeding difficulties
- attention problems, which may interfere with the patient's participation at mealtimes
- impulsive behaviors, which may lead to feeding difficulties (e.g., eating too fast and too much)
- drooling, which may cause the patient to be embarrassed
- coughing or throat clearing when the patient swallows food or liquids, which may result in pneumonia
- poor chewing skills, which may cause choking
- spillage of food and liquids falling outside of the lips, which may lead to weight loss or cause the patient embarrassment
- pocketing the food to the right or left side of the cheeks, which may cause choking
- untimely swallow (a loud clunking noise heard during the swallow), which may cause the patient to fatigue at mealtimes and lose weight
- increased congestion before or after meals, which may cause pneumonia

Staff Education 6
Inservice Resource 6.8

Compensatory Strategies for Safe Swallowing for Patients Who Have Suffered a CVA

The speech-language pathologist who evaluates the patient who has had a CVA may inform the nursing staff what compensatory strategies should be used to promote safe swallowing. The following recommendations may be useful:

- Position the patient in a 90-degree angle upright sitting position, with the feet flat on the floor or on the foot rests of the wheelchair.
- Assist the patient with tray setup, by offering only one plate of food and one liquid at a time to avoid overwhelming the patient.
- Give the patient verbal, visual, or tactile cues to:
  - ➢ take a small spoon of food at a time
  - ➢ chew, chew, and then swallow
  - ➢ place a spoon of food to the unaffected (and stronger) side of the mouth which will allow better chewing of food and chewing and swallowing food and liquid)
  - ➢ use a chin tuck for the swallow of food or liquids
  - ➢ use the tongue or a finger to sweep the lower and upper gums and the cheeks, to clear food or liquid that has gathered there
  - ➢ use a multiple dry swallow
  - ➢ push down when you swallow to create a hard swallow
- Give the patient verbal encouragement to eat and drink.
- Stroke the patient's throat upward toward the base of the tongue to help initiate a swallow reflex.

Staff Education 7

Swallowing Difficulties After Head Trauma

After experiencing head trauma, the patient may have one or more of the following difficulties:

- poor head and body positioning (the patient may have multiple fractures, may have very rigid muscle tone, or may be restless and agitated)
- bite reflex or a sucking reflex
- combative or impulsive behaviors
- feeding problems (patient eats too fast or too much)
- outbursts of inappropriate emotions
- verbalizations in the middle of a swallow
- attention deficits
- fatigue

Staff Education 7
Inservice Resource 6.9

Compensatory Strategies for Safe Swallowing for Patients with Head Trauma

With patients who have had a traumatic head injury, the speech-language pathologist may make the following recommendations for staff to promote safe swallowing:

- Position the patient in 90-degree angle sitting upright position with the feet flat on the floor or on the footrests of the wheelchair.
- Assist the patient with tray setup, presenting only one plate of food and one liquid at a time, to avoid overwhelming the patient.
- Give the patient verbal, visual, and tactile cues to:
  - ➢ slow down the rate of self-feeding
  - ➢ take a small spoon of food, not a large spoon
  - ➢ use the tongue or a finger to sweep the lower and upper gums and cheeks to clear food or liquid that has gathered there
  - ➢ "chew, chew, and swallow," thereby helping the patient remember to chew the food
- Stroke the patient's throat upward toward the base of the tongue to help the patient initiate a swallow reflex.
- Massage the patient's lower lip with a spoon or glass; when the lower lip relaxes, apply pressure and give the patient a spoon of food or sip of liquid.
- Instruct the patient to use a rubber-coated spoon.
- Instruct the patient not to bite down on the spoon.
- Tell the patient to open the mouth.
- Apply firm upward pressure under the lower jaw to release a bite reflex around a spoon, which is a counteraction release strategy.

Staff Education 6 & 7
Posttest

Swallowing After Trauma and CVA

1. The patient who has had a CVA may have problems seeing objects, people, and food to the affected side (right or left). This is called _____.

2. *True* or *False*: The patient who has had a CVA may cough or clear the throat while eating or drinking.

3. *True* or *False*: The patient who has had a CVA always has strong lip muscles; therefore, food or liquid spillage from the lips seldom occurs.

4. *True* or *False*: The patient who has had a CVA may pocket food in the cheek.

5. *True* or *False*: Telling the patient to slow down and eat only one spoonful at a time is considered unprofessional and therefore not recommended.

6. *True* or *False*: Stroke the patient's throat hard and with lots of pressure if you are trying to get the patient to start a swallow.

7. *True* or *False*: Putting only one plate of food and one liquid in front of a patient is a strategy used to get the patient to lose weight.

8. State two reasons why the patient who has had a traumatic head injury could be difficult to position.

   _____

   _____

9. *True* or *False*: The patient with a head trauma could have a bite reflex.

10. *True* or *False*: If the patient bites down on the spoon, the best thing to do is force it out of his or her mouth.

Staff Education 8

Physician Education on the Role of the Speech-Language Pathologist and Swallowing

Educating physicians about the specifics of dysphagia management is a slow and effortful process. A professional rapport and trust must be established with the physicians with whom the speech-language pathologist works. Physician education sometimes occurs when the physician asks a specific question about the patient's swallowing abilities. The speech-language pathologist can assist physicians in managing their patients with dysphagia in the following ways:

- Through educating physicians on the role of the speech-language pathologist in assessing and managing swallowing disorders in patients they serve
- Through the clinical bedside evaluation
- Through the modified barium videofluoroscopic swallow study
- Through dysphagia treatment for the patient
- Through developing safe swallowing programs for their patients

Staff Education 8
Inservice Resource 6.10
Educating the Physician

Target Staff: Physicians in charge of patients with dysphagia

Purpose: To educate physicians on intervention goals for dysphagia and the roles, responsibilities, and expertise of speech-language pathologists in assessing and treating patients with dysphagia

Objectives: By the end of the inservice session, the participants will appreciate the following:

Dysphagia Intervention

Dysphagia intervention has the following goals:

- Preventing and decreasing the risk for aspiration, pneumonia, or choking
- Decreasing the patient's length of stay and additional complications
- Establishing a safe oral feeding program for the patient
- Improving quality of life for the patient

The Clinical Bedside Evaluation

The speech-language pathologist can obtain the following information from the clinical bedside evaluation:

- how the patient manages and forms a bolus
- how the vocal folds are adducting to protect the larynx
- how the laryngeal muscles are moving to help in the swallow
- what texture of food and liquid the patient can tolerate
- whether audible signs of aspiration (e.g., wet or gurgly vocal quality, coughing or throat clearing) are present on food or liquid ingestion

Modified Barium Videofluoroscopic Swallow Study (MBVSS)

Both the speech-language pathologist and the radiologist perform the MBVSS. The speech-language pathologist obtains the following information from the MBVSS:

- confirms or rules out aspiration
- determines the types of textures of food or liquid the patient can consume without aspirating
- determines if there are compensatory or positioning techniques that can be used to allow the patient to eat and drink without aspiration
- determines whether a patient can continue to eat or drink by mouth

Dysphagia Treatment for the Patient

The speech-language pathologist provides dysphagia treatment to:

- improve the strength of the oral, pharyngeal, and laryngeal musculature
- advance the patient's diet to the least restrictive food and liquid consistencies

The Development of Safe Swallowing Programs

The speech-language pathologist may:

- develop safe swallowing programs for the patient in the hospital, in skilled nursing facility, and in the patient's home
- establish specific compensatory strategies and postures for the patient and families to consider
- present and discuss the options available to the patient with severe swallowing difficulties
- discuss alternate means of feeding (e.g., tube feedings) and their pros and cons with the patient and the family

Staff Education 8
Posttest

Educating the Physician

1. *True* or *False*: Intervention for dysphagia by a speech-language pathologist may prevent and decrease the risk of aspiration or choking.

2. *True* or *False*: Collaboration with a speech-language pathologist may decrease the patient's length of stay and additional complications at the hospital.

3. *True* or *False*: A speech-language pathologist may not recommend a diet consistency for a patient; this should be done by a registered dietitian.

4. *True* or *False*: A speech-language pathologist may not recommend tube feedings for a patient.

5. *True* or *False*: A radiologist together with a speech-language pathologist may confirm and rule out aspiration.

6. The speech-language pathologist may evaluate and treat your patient for dysphagia:
   A. Without a physician order from you.
   B. Only with a physician order from you.
   C. None of the above.

7. The clinical bedside swallow evaluation by a speech language pathologist can determine whether:
   A. The patient has pneumonia and needs to be hospitalized.
   B. Audible signs of aspiration on food and liquids are present when the patient swallows.
   C. None of the above.

8. To develop a safe swallow program, the speech-language pathologist may provide dysphagia treatment in:
   A. Acute care hospitals, skilled nursing facilities, and the patient's home.
   B. Acute care hospitals only.
   C. None of the above.

9. Which of the following patients should be referred by the speech-language pathologist for a modified barium videofluoroscopic swallow study?
   A. All patients who undergo a clinical bedside swallow evaluation.
   B. Patients who meet the criteria to safely undergo a modified barium videofluoroscopic swallow study.
   C. None of the above.

10. The speech-language pathologist should provide training in safe swallowing techniques and postures to
    A. The patient.
    B. The patient's family.
    C. The nurse.
    D. All of the above.

Section 7

Therapy Resources for Patients and Nursing Staff and Posting

This section presents various therapy resources, in both English and Spanish. These resources can be discussed by the clinician with the family or nursing staff, depending on the patient's specific swallowing difficulty. The clinician may print them out and give them to the patient, members of the patient's family, and nursing staff or post them in appropriate places (e.g., the patient's room).

Therapy resources are provided for the following topics:

☐ Symptoms of Dysphagia

☐ Dysphagia Precautions

☐ Choking Precautions

☐ Choking on Pills or Medications

☐ NPO—Nothing by Mouth

☐ Patient Environment at Mealtimes

☐ Various patient positionings during and after mealtimes (multiple topics)

☐ Liquid Consistency

☐ Diet Consistency

☐ Safe swallowing instructions (multiple topics)

☐ Chewing Problems and Solutions

☐ Food Management Problems

☐ Difficulty Removing Food from Utensils

☐ Difficulty with Food Sticking to the Roof of the Mouth

☐ Holding Food Inside the Mouth

☐ Food Is Falling Outside the Patient's Mouth

☐ The Patient Will Not Open the Mouth

☐ The Patient with a Bite Reflex

☐ The Patient Has Oral Thrush or Sores in the Mouth

☐ Working with the Patient Who Has Dementia

☐ The Patient Who Has Had A Stroke

☐ The Patient's Oral Care

Therapy Resource 7.1a (English)

Symptoms of Dysphagia

☐ The patient has food or liquid falling outside of the mouth.

☐ The patient has food or liquid that stays inside the mouth even after swallowing.

☐ The patient has food or liquid that gets stuck inside of the cheek.

☐ The patient coughs before swallowing when food or liquid is inside the mouth.

☐ The patient coughs while eating or drinking.

☐ The patient coughs after eating foods or drinking liquids.

☐ The patient clears the throat while drinking liquids or eating food.

☐ The patient clears the throat after drinking liquids or eating food.

☐ The patient chokes while eating food or drinking liquids.

☐ The patient chokes after eating foods or drinking liquids.

☐ The patient makes an effortful face while swallowing food or liquid.

☐ The patient has a lot of phlegm and congestion after eating food or drinking liquids.

☐ The patient complains of food or liquid getting stuck in the throat.

☐ The patient complains of pain in the throat area with increased difficulty swallowing.

☐ The patient has a wet- or "gurgly"-sounding voice after swallowing foods or liquids.

☐ The patient has a fever.

Therapy Resource 7.1b (Spanish)

Síntomas de Disfagia

☐ El paciente tiene comida o líquido que se le sale de la boca.

☐ El paciente tiene comida o líquido que se le queda dentro de la boca después de que traga.

☐ El paciente tiene comida o líquido que se atora dentro de la mejilla.

☐ El paciente tose antes de tragar cuando tiene comida o líquido dentro de la boca.

☐ El paciente tose cuando come o toma.

☐ El paciente tose después de tragar comida o tomar líquidos.

☐ El paciente se aclara la voz mientras que traga líquidos o come comida.

☐ El paciente se aclara la voz después de tragar líquidos o come comida.

☐ El paciente se ahoga cuando traga comida o líquidos.

☐ El paciente se ahoga después de que traga comida o líquidos.

☐ El paciente hace cara de esfuerzo cuando traga comida o liquido.

☐ El paciente tiene mucha flema y ahoguijo después de que traga comida o líquidos.

☐ El paciente se queja que la comida o el líquido se le atora en la garganta.

☐ El paciente se queja de dolor en la garganta con más dificultad cuando traga.

☐ El paciente tiene voz mojada y borboteada después de que traga comida o líquidos.

☐ El paciente tiene fiebre.

Therapy Resource 7.2a (English)

Dysphagia Precautions

Aspiration Precautions

☐ The head of the patient's bed should be up and at a 25-degree angle at all times, to decrease the risk of aspiration.

☐ The patient should remain sitting up for at least 30 minutes after eating or drinking. This will decrease the risk of aspiration and reflux.

☐ Listen for the wet, gurgly sounds of increased congestion and phlegm during breathing or talking.

☐ If the patient may have aspirated, ask the patient to cough and clear the throat, until the patient's chest/throat sounds clear.

☐ If congestion continues, it may be necessary to suction the patient's airway.

☐ The patient's temperature should be monitored for the next 24 to 72 hours.

☐ The patient's lungs should be checked every day.

☐ The liquid and diet consistency must be what the speech pathologist recommended to decrease the risk of aspiration.

☐ Avoid letting patient use a straw, because it causes the liquids too move to quickly into the patient's mouth.

☐ The patient should avoid tilting the head back while swallowing.

☐ The patient should be in a 90-degree angle sitting position for all meals.

☐ Avoid distractions. Have the patient concentrate on swallowing.

☐ Instruct the patient to use a chin tuck to swallow, if needed.

Therapy Resource 7.2b (Spanish)

Precauciones de Disfagia

Precauciones de Aspiración

☐ La cabecera de la cama del paciente debe estar hacia arriba en un ángulo de 25-grados a todo tiempo, para disminuir el riesgo de aspiración.

☐ El paciente debe de mantenerse sentado a menos de 30 minutos, después de comer o tragar. Esto es para disminuir el riesgo de aspiración o reflejo.

☐ Escuche por sonidos mojados o borboteados de ahoguijo y flema, mientras que respira o habla.

☐ Si el paciente puede ser aspirado, pídale al paciente que tosa y se aclare la voz, hasta que el paciente se oiga claro.

☐ Si la congestión continua, tal vez es necesario aspirar la vía aérea del paciente.

☐ La temperatura del paciente debe ser comprobada por los siguientes 24 a 72 horas.

☐ La condición de los pulmones del paciente puede ser comprobada diaria.

☐ La dieta y consistencia de los líquidos debe ser lo que la terapista de habla y lenguaje recomendó para disminuir el riesgo de aspiración.

☐ Evite que el paciente use popote, porque con el popote los líquidos se sorben muy rápido a la boca del paciente.

☐ El paciente debe evitar de inclinar la cabeza hacia atrás mientras que el paciente traga.

☐ El paciente debe de estar sentado derecho en un ángulo de 90-grados cada vez que come.

☐ Evite distracciones.

☐ El paciente debe de concentrar en su tragar.

☐ Enséñele al paciente que debe poner la barbilla hacia el pecho cuando trague.

Therapy Resource 7.3a (English)

Choking Precautions

☐ The patient must be in a 90-degree angle sitting position while drinking or eating.

☐ The rate of feeding or drinking must be slow. Give the patient verbal cues such as "Take one drink at a time."

☐ The amount of food or liquid placed in the patient's mouth must be small, to decrease the risk of choking.

☐ Have the patient concentrate on eating and swallowing. Avoid distractions while the patient is eating.

☐ Avoid asking the patient questions when he or she has food or liquid in the mouth.

☐ The patient should avoid tilting the head back while eating.

☐ The patient may complain of food "getting stuck" in the throat.

☐ The patient may look frightened and not be able to speak.

☐ The patient may grab the throat area.

☐ Allow the patient plenty of time to eat.

☐ Have patient lower the chin to the chest for each swallow.

☐ Avoid foods that are tough or hard to chew.

☐ If foods are dry, add gravy or sauce to hold the food together. This will improve the swallow transit for the patient.

☐ Get training for cardiopulmonary resuscitation (CPR).

☐ Know how to apply the Heimlich maneuver, if needed.

Therapy Resource 7.3b (Spanish)

Precauciones de Ahogo

☐ El paciente debe de estar sentado derecho en un ángulo de 90-grados cuando toma o come.

☐ El ritmo de comer o tragar debe ser despacio. Dale al paciente una señal verbal: "Tome un trago a la vez."

☐ La cantidad de comida o líquido que se pone en la boca del paciente debe ser pequeña, para disminuir el riesgo de ahogo.

☐ El paciente tiene que concentrar en comer y tragar. Evite distracciones mientras que el paciente come.

☐ Evite preguntándole preguntas al paciente, mientras que el paciente tiene comida o líquido en la boca.

☐ El paciente debe de evitar de inclinar la cabeza hacia atrás mientras que come.

☐ El paciente tal vez se queje que la comida "se le atora" en la garganta.

☐ El paciente quizás se mire asustado y no podrá hablar.

☐ Este paciente quizás se agarre la garganta.

☐ Permítale bastante tiempo al paciente para que coma.

☐ El paciente debe de poner la barbilla hacia abajo sobre el pecho para cada trago.

☐ Evite comidas que son duras y dificultosas para masticar.

☐ Si la comida esta seca, póngale jugo o salsa, para que la comida se retenga junta. Esto mejorara el transito del tragar.

☐ Adquirí entrenamiento de resucitación cardiopulmonar.

☐ Debe de saber Aplicar el maniobro de Heimlich, si es necesario.

Therapy Resource 7.4a (English)

Choking on Pills or Medications

☐ Have the patient sit up to swallow pills.

☐ Offer one pill at a time.

☐ Give pills or medications with applesauce.

☐ Open or crush all pills or medications and give with applesauce (check with pharmacist first).

☐ Request all medications in liquid form (if the patient is on thick liquids, thicken the liquid medications to the appropriate consistency).

Therapy Resource 7.4b (Spanish)

Ahogo con Pastillas o Medicaciones

☐ El paciente se debe de sentar derecho para tragar las pastillas.

☐ Ofrezca una pastilla a la vez.

☐ De las pastillas o medicaciones con manzana molida.

☐ Abra o machuque todas las pastillas o medicaciones y déselas con manzana molida primero hable con el farmacéutico).

☐ Suplique que todas las medicaciones sean en forma de líquido (si el paciente recibe líquidos espesos, los medicamentos de líquido se deben espesar a la consistencia apropiada).

Therapy Resource 7.5a (English)

NPO

NOTHING
BY MOUTH

Therapy Resource 7.5b (Spanish)

NADA

POR

LA BOCA

Therapy Resource 7.6a (English)

Patient Environment at Mealtimes

THE FOLLOWING ENVIRONMENTAL PROCEDURES SHOULD BE IMPLEMENTED IN THE PATIENT'S HOME ENVIRONMENT:

☐ The area where the patient eats should be quiet and free from distractions (e.g., TV or radio).

☐ The environment should be structured and consistent (e.g., same seating arrangement).

☐ The family members should not encourage talking while the patient is eating.

El Ambiente del Paciente a la Hora de Comer

LOS SIGUIENTES PROCEDIMIENTOS AMBIENTALES SE DEBEN DE LLEVAR A CABO EN EL AMBIENTE DEL HOGAR DEL PACIENTE:

☐ El área donde come el paciente debe de estar en silencio y libre de distracciones (e.g., televisión o radio).

☐ El ambiente debe de ser firme con pocos cambios (e.g., el mismo lugar para sentarse).

☐ Los miembros de la familia no deben de animar que se hable mientras que el paciente coma.

Therapy Resource 7.7a (English)

Patient Position During Mealtimes

PATIENT SHOULD BE SITTING IN A 90° UPRIGHT POSITION AT ALL MEALTIMES

Posición del Paciente Durante la Hora de Comer

EL PACIENTE DEBE ESTAR SENTADO DERECHO EN POSICIÓN DE 90° A TODA HORA DE COMIDA

Therapy Resource 7.8a (English)

Patient Position After Each Meal

PATIENT SHOULD BE SITTING IN A 90° POSITION FOR 30 MINUTES AFTER MEALTIMES

Therapy Resource 7.8b (Spanish)

Posición del Paciente Después de Cada Comida

EL PACIENTE DEBE DE ESTAR SENTADO EN POSICIÓN DE 90° POR 30 MINUTOS DESPUÉS DE TODAS LAS COMIDAS

Therapy Resource 7.9a (English)

Patient's Head Position During Mealtimes

PATIENT SHOULD KEEP HEAD IN A STRAIGHT POSITION DURING MEALTIMES

(THE PATIENT SHOULD NOT TILT THE HEAD BACK)

Posición de la Cabeza del Paciente Durante la Hora de la Comida

EL PACIENTE DEBE DE MANTENER SU CABEZA EN UNA POSICIÓN DERECHA DURANTE LA HORA DE LA COMIDA

(EL PACIENTE NO DEBE DE INCLINAR SU CABEZA HACIA ATRÁS)

Therapy Resource 7.10a (English)

Patient's Foot Position During Mealtimes

PATIENT'S FEET SHOULD REMAIN ON THE FLOOR OR FOOT REST DURING MEALTIMES

Therapy Resource 7.10b (Spanish)

Posición de los Pies del Paciente Durante la Hora de la Comida

LOS PIES DEL PACIENTE DEBEN DE MANTENERSE EN EL PISO O EN EL REPOSA PIES DURANTE LA HORA DE LA COMIDA

Therapy Resource 7.11a (English)

Checklist for Patient's Head Position During Mealtimes

USE ONLY THE INSTRUCTIONS THAT ARE CHECKED OFF FOR THE PATIENT

☐ The patient should put the head down to the chest before swallowing food.

☐ The patient should put the head down to the chest before swallowing liquids.

☐ The patient should turn the head to the left before swallowing food or liquid.

☐ The patient should turn the head to the right before swallowing food or liquid.

☐ The patient should turn the head to the right and put the chin down toward the chest before swallowing food or liquid.

☐ The patient should turn the head to the left and put the chin down before swallowing food or liquid.

continues

Therapy Resource 7.11a (English), *continued*

Checklist for Patient's Head Position During Mealtimes

☐ The patient should take a bite of food and swallow using a hard effortful swallow.

☐ The patient should take a drink of liquid and swallow using a hard effortful swallow.

☐ The patient should take a bite of food and swallow and then swallow again with no food in the mouth.

☐ The patient should take a sip of liquid and swallow and then swallow again with no liquid in the mouth.

☐ The patient should take a bite of food and then a drink of liquid throughout the meal.

☐ The patient should place the food to the right side of the mouth and chew.

☐ The patient should place the food to the left side of the mouth and chew.

☐ The patient should use a straw to drink liquids.

☐ The patient should not use a straw to drink liquids.

☐ The patient should use a spoon to drink liquids.

Therapy Resource 7.11b (Spanish)

Lista de Marcar la Posición de la Cabeza del Paciente Durante la Hora de la Comida

USE SOLO LAS INSTRUCCIONES QUE SON MARCADAS PARA EL PACIENTE

☐ El paciente debe poner su cabeza hacia abajo en su pecho antes de tragar comida.

☐ El paciente debe poner su cabeza hacia abajo en su pecho antes de tragar líquidos.

☐ El paciente debe voltear su cabeza a la izquierda antes de tragar comida o líquido.

☐ El paciente debe voltear su cabeza a la derecha antes de tragar comida o líquido.

☐ El paciente debe voltear su cabeza a la derecha y poner su barbilla hacia abajo en su pecho antes de tragar comida o líquido.

☐ El paciente debe voltear su cabeza a la izquierda y poner su barbilla hacia abajo en su pecho antes de tragar comida o líquido.

continúa

Therapy Resource 7.11b (Spanish), *continuado*

Lista de Marcar la Posición de la Cabeza del Paciente Durante la Hora de la Comida

☐ El paciente debe agarrar un bocado de comida y tragarlo usando un gran esfuerzo en el tragar.

☐ El paciente debe tomar un trago de líquido usando un gran esfuerzo en el tragar.

☐ El paciente debe agarrar un bocado de comida y tragárselo y luego tragar otra vez sin comida en la boca.

☐ El paciente debe tomar un sorbo de líquido y tragárselo y luego tragar otra vez sin líquido en la boca.

☐ El paciente debe tragar un bocado de comida y luego un trago de líquido durante toda la comida.

☐ El paciente debe poner la comida al lado derecho de la boca y masticarla.

☐ El paciente se debe poner la comida al lado izquierdo de la boca y masticarla.

☐ El paciente debe usar un popote para tomar sus líquidos.

☐ El paciente no debe usar popote para tomar sus líquidos.

☐ El paciente debe usar una cuchara para tomar sus líquidos.

Therapy Resource 7.12a (English)

Clinician's Checklist for Patient's General Position

USE ONLY THE POSITIONING STRATEGIES THAT ARE CHECKED OFF BY THE CLINICIAN:

☐ The patient should be positioned so that the hips, knees, and ankles form a 90° angle.

☐ The patient's feet should be well supported during mealtimes.

☐ The patient should sit with the back straight in the chair (this will reduce leaning to either side).

Lista de Marcar del Clínico para la Posición General del Paciente

USE SOLAMENTE LAS ESTRATEGIAS PARA POSICIONAR QUE ESTÁN MARCADAS POR LA TERAPISTA:

☐ El paciente debe estar posicionado para que las caderas, rodillas, y tobillos formen un ángulo de 90-grados.

☐ Los pies del paciente deben estar bien soportados durante la hora de la comida.

☐ El paciente se debe de sentar con su espalda derecha en la silla (esto reduce que se incline por los lados).

Therapy Resource 7.13a (English)

Liquid Consistency

THE PATIENT HAS TO DRINK:

☐ PUDDING-THICKENED LIQUIDS

☐ HONEY-THICKENED LIQUIDS

☐ NECTAR-THICKENED LIQUIDS

☐ REGULAR LIQUIDS

Consistencia de Líquidos

EL PACIENTE TIENE QUE TOMAR:

☐ LÍQUIDOS A PUDÍN

☐ LÍQUIDOS A MIEL

☐ LÍQUIDOS A NÉCTAR

☐ LÍQUIDOS REGULARES

Therapy Resource 7.14a (English)

Diet Consistency

THE PATIENT HAS
TO EAT:

☐ LIQUID PUREED CONSISTENCY

☐ PUREED CONSISTENCY

☐ FINELY CHOPPED CONSISTENCY

☐ MECHANICAL SOFT CONSISTENCY

☐ REGULAR CONSISTENCY

Therapy Resource 7.14b (Spanish)

Consistencia de Dieta

EL PACIENTE TIENE QUE COMER:

☐ CONSISTENCIA LICUADA POCO DENSA

☐ CONSISTENCIA LICUADA

☐ CONSISTENCIA CORTADA FINA

☐ CONSISTENCIA CORTADA EN PEDAZOS PEQUEÑOS

☐ CONSISTENCIA REGULAR

Therapy Resource 7.15a (English)

Safe Swallowing Instruction 1

THE PATIENT SHOULD EAT ONLY ONE TEASPOON OF FOOD AT A TIME

Therapy Resource 7.15b (Spanish)

Instrucción para el Tragar Seguro 1

EL PACIENTE DEBE DE COMER SOLAMENTE UNA CUCHARADA DE COMIDA A LA VEZ

Therapy Resource 7.16a (English)

Safe Swallowing Instruction 2

THE PATIENT SHOULD SWALLOW THE FOOD PLACED IN THE MOUTH BEFORE TAKING ANOTHER SPOON OF FOOD

EL PACIENTE DEBE DE TRAGAR LA COMIDA QUE TIENE EN SU BOCA ANTES DE TOMAR OTRA CUCHARADA DE COMIDA

Therapy Resource 7.17a (English)

Safe Swallowing Instruction 3

THE PATIENT SHOULD EAT SLOWLY

Therapy Resource 7.17b (Spanish)

Instrucción para el Tragar Seguro 3

EL PACIENTE DEBE COMER DESPACIO

Therapy Resource 7.18a (English)

Safe Swallowing Instruction 4

THE PATIENT SHOULD TAKE ONE SIP OF LIQUID AT A TIME

Therapy Resource 7.18b (Spanish)

Instrucción para el Tragar Seguro 4

EL PACIENTE DEBE TOMAR UN SORBO DE LÍQUIDO A LA VEZ

Therapy Resource 7.19a (English)

Safe Swallowing Instruction 5

THE PATIENT SHOULD DRINK LIQUIDS SLOWLY

Therapy Resource 7.19b (Spanish)

Instrucción para el Tragar Seguro 5

EL PACIENTE DEBE TOMAR LOS LÍQUIDOS DESPACIO

Therapy Resource 7.20a (English)

Safe Swallowing Instruction 6

THE PATIENT SHOULD TAKE ONE SMALL SIP AT A TIME

Therapy Resource 7.20b (Spanish)

Instrucción para el Tragar Seguro 6

EL PACIENTE DEBE TOMAR UN SORBO PEQUEÑO A LA VEZ

Therapy Resource 7.21a (English)

Safe Swallowing Instruction 7

THE PATIENT SHOULD EAT ONE SMALL TEASPOON OF FOOD AT A TIME

(PATIENT SHOULD NOT USE A LARGE SPOON TO EAT)

EL PACIENTE DEBE DE COMER UNA CUCHARADA PEQUEÑA DE COMIDA A LA VEZ

(EL PACIENTE NO DEBE COMER CON UNA CUCHARA GRANDE)

Therapy Resource 7.22a (English)

Chewing Problems and Solutions

☐ If the patient wears dentures to eat, the clinician should make sure that the patient has the dentures inside the mouth before eating.

☐ The caregiver should make sure the patient's dentures fit securely.

☐ The caregiver should make sure that denture adhesive has been applied to the patient's dentures.

☐ The caregiver should give the patient verbal cues such as "Chew, chew, chew, and then swallow."

☐ The caregiver should ask the patient to open the mouth after swallowing to make sure the mouth is clear of food and liquid.

☐ The caregiver should place only small amounts of food inside the patient's mouth at a time.

☐ The caregiver should give the patient verbal cues to use the tongue to sweep the sides of the cheeks with the tongue to collect food or liquid that has remained after the swallow.

continues

Therapy Resource 7.22a (English), *continued*

Chewing Problems and Solutions

☐ The caregiver should show the patient how to sweep the cheeks and gums with the tongue by performing this maneuver on himself/herself.

☐ The caregiver should touch the patient's cheeks with a finger to remind the patient to do the tongue sweep after the swallow.

☐ The caregiver should place the food on side of the mouth that is the strongest (__right __left).

☐ The caregiver should place a mirror in front of the patient while the patient is eating so the patient can see if food or liquid is getting stuck inside the cheeks after the swallow.

☐ The caregiver should help the patient with oral hygiene after the swallow. This should include the following:

○ Instruct the patient to rinse and spit.

○ Use a Toothette to remove food remaining inside the mouth if the patient is unable to do this.

Therapy Resource 7.22b (Spanish)

Problemas de Masticar y las Soluciones

☐ Si el paciente usa dentadura postiza para comer, la terapista debe estar segura que el paciente trae su dentadura puesta en la boca antes de comer.

☐ El asistente debe asegurarse que la dentadura le quede bien al paciente.

☐ El asistente debe asegurarse que la dentadura del paciente tiene adhesiva para dentaduras.

☐ El asistente debe darle señales verbales al paciente como ("Mastique, mastique, mastique y luego trague").

☐ El asistente debe pedirle al paciente que abra la boca después de que trague, para asegurarse que no hay comida o líquido en la boca.

☐ El asistente solo debe poner cantidades pequeñas de comida a la vez en la boca del paciente.

☐ El asistente debe darle al paciente señales verbales para que con su lengua limpie la comida o líquidos que se hayan adherido dentro de su boca después del trago.

continúa

Therapy Resource 7.22b (Spanish), *continuado*

Problemas de Masticar y las Soluciones

☐ El asistente debe enseñarle al paciente como limpiar las mejillas y las encías con la lengua llevando a cabo esta maniobra en si mismo.

☐ El asistente debe tocar las mejillas del paciente con su dedo para recordarle que use la lengua para limpiar la boca después de tragar.

☐ El asistente debe poner la comida en el lado de la boca que esta más fuerte (derecho izquierdo).

☐ El asistente debe poner un espejo enfrente del paciente mientras que el paciente come para que el paciente pueda ver si comida o líquido se atoro en las mejillas después del tragar.

☐ El asistente debe ayudarle al paciente con la higiene bucal después del tragar. Esto debe de incluir lo siguiente:

   ○ Instruya al paciente para que se enjuague su boca y escupa.

   ○ Use una esponjita para quitar la comida de adentro de la boca del paciente si es algo que el paciente no puede hacer.

Therapy Resource 7.23a (English)

Food Management Problems

☐ The caregiver should make sure the patient's food is moist.

☐ The caregiver should use gravy or sauce on all meats.

☐ The caregiver should make sure that the patient does not mix solid foods with liquids in the same mouthful.

☐ The caregiver should make sure the patient swallows the food completely and then offers the patient something to drink.

☐ The caregiver should encourage the patient to take full teaspoon-size bites.

Therapy Resource 7.23b (Spanish)

Problemas Manejando la Comida

☐ El asistente debe asegurarse que la comida del paciente este húmeda.

☐ El asiente debe usar jugo o salsas sobre las carnes.

☐ El asistente debe asegurarse que el paciente no mezcle la comida con los líquidos en el mismo bocado.

☐ El asistente debe asegurarse que el paciente se trague la comida completamente y luego de ofrecerle algo para tomar.

☐ El asistente debe animar al paciente para que se dé una cucharada a la vez.

Therapy Resource 7.24a (English)

Difficulty Removing Food From Utensils

☐ The caregiver should place food at the tip of the spoon.

☐ The caregiver should present the food to the front of the patient with the spoon below eye level.

☐ The caregiver should place the spoon in the patient's mouth and apply firm pressure on the middle of the patient's tongue.

☐ The caregiver should give the patient verbal cues, such as "Close your lips around the spoon and remove the food that is on the spoon."

☐ The caregiver should remove the spoon as soon as the patient's lips begin to close around the spoon (making sure not to scrape the patient's upper teeth with the spoon).

☐ The caregiver should serve the patient as many finger foods as possible to strengthen the lip seal.

☐ The caregiver should never use a spoon that is larger than a teaspoon.

Therapy Resource 7.24b (Spanish)

Dificultad Quitando la Comida de los Utensilios

☐ El asistente debe poner la comida en la punta de la cuchara.

☐ El asistente debe presentar la comida frente al paciente con la cuchara abajo del nivel de los ojos del paciente.

☐ El asistente debe poner la cuchara en la boca del paciente y aplicar presión firme en medio de la lengua del paciente.

☐ El asistente debe darle al paciente señales verbales como: "Cierre los labios alrededor de la cuchara y quite la comida que está en la cuchara."

☐ El asistente debe quitar la cuchara cuando los labios del paciente comiencen a cerrar alrededor de la cuchara (asegúrese de no raspar los dientes de arriba con la cuchara).

☐ El asistente debe servirle al paciente todas las comidas posibles que son fáciles para comer con los dedos para fortalecer la sellada de los labios.

☐ El asistente nunca debe usar una cuchara que es más grande que una cucharilla.

Therapy Resource 7.25a (English)

Difficulty with Food Sticking to Roof of Mouth

☐ The caregiver should give the patient verbal cues: "Use your tongue and sweep the roof of your mouth with it. This will remove the food from the roof of your mouth."

☐ The caregiver should give the patient a visual cue by performing this maneuver himself/herself while the patient watches.

☐ The caregiver should have the patient open the mouth after swallowing and check to see if the food and liquid are cleared from the mouth.

☐ The caregiver should remove food or liquid that is left in the mouth after the swallow with a Toothette, to prevent the patient from choking.

☐ The caregiver should give the patient a mirror so the patient can check to see if there is any food left on the roof of the mouth.

☐ The caregiver should have the patient take a bite of food and then a drink of liquid, to clear the food from the roof of the mouth.

☐ The caregiver should give the patient food that has gravy or sauce on it.

Therapy Resource 7.25b (Spanish)

Dificultad con la Comida que se Pega en el Paladar

☐ El asistente debe darle al paciente señales verbales ("Use su lengua, limpie el paladar con ella. Esto removerá la comida del paladar).

☐ El asistente debe darle al paciente una señal visual llevando a cabo esta maniobra en sí mismo mientras que el paciente observa.

☐ El asistente debe pedirle al paciente que abra la boca después de que traga para revisar si la comida o líquido se limpiaron de la boca.

☐ El asistente debe quitar la comida o líquido que se ha quedado en la boca después de tragar con una esponjita o un depresor de lengua para evitar que se ahogue el paciente.

☐ El asistente debe darle al paciente un espejo para que el paciente revise si quedo comida en el paladar.

☐ El asistente debe dejar al paciente tomar un bocado de comida y luego un trago de líquido para que se limpie la comida del paladar.

☐ El asistente debe darle al paciente comida que tiene jugo o salsa.

Therapy Resource 7.26a (English)

Holding Food Inside the Mouth

☐ The caregiver should place one teaspoon in the patient's mouth at a time.

☐ The caregiver should ask the patient to open the mouth to see if the food or liquid has been swallowed before the next spoon is introduced to the patient.

☐ The caregiver should give the patient verbal cues, such as "Chew your food and then swallow."

☐ The caregiver should place the fingers under the patient's chin and gently stroke downward, to help initiate the patient's swallow reflex.

☐ The caregiver should place a spoon or glass to the patient's lower lip and press down gently against the lip.

☐ The caregiver should press slightly downward on the tongue so when the spoon is removed from the patient's mouth to help stimulate a swallow reflex.

☐ The caregiver should show the patient the next spoonful of food or cup of liquid, when the patient is holding food or liquid inside the mouth. This reminds the patient to swallow because the patient has to get ready for the next bite of food or drink of liquid.

☐ The caregiver should place the spoon in ice water between bites of food. The cold sensation should help trigger the swallow reflex.

☐ The caregiver should have the patient alternate a bite of food with a swallow of liquid.

Therapy Resource 7.26b (Spanish)

Reteniendo la Comida en la Boca

☐ El asistente debe poner una cucharada a la vez en la boca del paciente.

☐ El asistente debe pedirle al paciente que abra la boca para ver si la comida o líquido fue tragada antes de que le dé la siguiente cucharada.

☐ El asistente debe darle al paciente señales verbales como: "Mastique su comida y luego tragué."

☐ El asistente debe poner sus dedos abajo de la barbilla del paciente y ablandar el área para abajo para ayudar al paciente con el comienzo del tragar.

☐ El asistente debe poner la cuchara o el vaso en el labio de abajo del paciente y apretar suavemente contra el labio.

☐ El ayudante debe presionar ligeramente hacia abajo en la lengua cuando la cuchara es removida de la boca del paciente para estimular el reflejo del tragar.

☐ El asistente debe enseñarle al paciente la siguiente cucharada de comida o taza de líquido cuando el paciente esta reteniendo la comida o líquido en su boca. Esto le recuerda al paciente que necesita tragar lo que tiene en su boca para estar listo para el siguiente bocado de comida o trago de líquido.

☐ El asistente debe poner la cuchara en agua helada entre bocados de comida. La sensación fría ayudará a funcionar el reflejo de tragar.

☐ El asistente debe decirle al paciente que alterne un bocado de comida con un sorbo de líquido.

Therapy Resource 7.27a (English)

Food Is Falling Outside the Patient's Mouth

☐ The caregiver should have the patient use a straw for liquids (if the patient is able to suck).

☐ The caregiver should give the patient a special cup with a lid that has a spout for drinking liquids.

☐ The caregiver should place the food in the middle of the patient's tongue, giving the patient verbal cues: "Keep your lips closed, chew, and swallow."

Therapy Resource 7.27b (Spanish)

Comida que se Sale de la Boca

☐ El asistente debe dejar que el paciente use un popote para los líquidos (sí el paciente pueda sorber).

☐ El asistente debe darle al paciente una taza especial con tapadera que tiene pico para tomar líquidos.

☐ El asistente debe poner la comida en medio de la lengua del paciente dándole al paciente una señal verbal: "Mantenga sus labios cerrados, mastique y tragué."

Therapy Resource 7.28a (English)

The Patient Will Not Open The Mouth

☐ The caregiver should give the patient verbal cues, such as "Open your mouth."

☐ Caregivers can give visual cues by opening their own mouth while the patient watches.

☐ The caregiver should touch the patient's lips with a little bit of food or liquid from the spoon to stimulate mouth opening.

☐ The caregiver should apply gentle pressure down on the patient's chin to open the mouth.

☐ The caregiver can apply gentle downward pressure on the lower lip with a spoon or glass. This may encourage mouth opening.

Therapy Resource 7.28b (Spanish)

El Paciente que no Abre la Boca

☐ El asistente debe darle al paciente señales verbales, como, "Abra la boca."

☐ Los asistentes pueden darle señales visuales por medio de abrir su propia boca mientras que el paciente observa.

☐ El asistente debe tocar los labios del paciente con poca comida o líquido para estimular abertura de la boca.

☐ El asistente debe aplicar presión suavemente sobre la barbilla del paciente para que se abra la boca.

☐ El asistente debe aplicar presión suavemente en el labio de abajo con la cuchara o el vaso. Esto quizás anime al paciente par que abra la boca.

Therapy Resource 7.29a (English)

The Patient with a Bite Reflex

☐ The caregiver should not let the patient use plastic utensils (These are dangerous because they can break inside the patient's mouth.)

☐ The caregiver should provide rubber-coated metal spoons for the patient to use.

☐ The caregiver should verbally instruct the patient "Do not bite down on the spoon."

☐ The caregiver should place a spoon of food into the side of the patient's mouth and tell the patient: "Use your tongue to get the food from the side of your mouth."

Therapy Resource 7.29b (Spanish)

El Paciente con el Reflejo de Morder

☐ El asistente no debe dejar que el paciente use utensilios de plástico (estos son peligrosos porque se pueden quebrar dentro de la boca del paciente).

☐ El asistente debe proveer cucharas cubiertas con vinilo para que coma el paciente.

☐ El asistente debe instruir verbalmente al paciente: "No muerda la cuchara."

☐ El asistente debe poner una cuchara de comida dentro del lado de la boca del paciente y decirle al paciente: "Use su lengua para agarrar la comida del lado de su boca."

Therapy Resource 7.30a (English)

The Patient Has Oral Thrush or Sores in the Mouth

☐ The patient should avoid sour or acidic food or liquids (e.g., orange juice or grapefruit juice).

☐ The caregiver should serve foods cold or at room temperature. Do not serve hot food, as this will irritate the condition of the mouth.

☐ The caregiver should have the patient alternate one bite of food with a sip of liquid.

Therapy Resource 7.30b (Spanish)

El Paciente Que Tiene Algodoncillo o Granos en la Boca

☐ El paciente debe evitar comidas o líquidos agrios o con ácido (por ejemplo, jugo de naranja o toronja).

☐ El asistente debe servir comidas frías. No sirva comidas calientes porque esto irrita más la condición de la boca.

☐ El asistente debe dejar que el paciente alterne un bocado de comida con un sorbo de líquido.

Therapy Resource 7.31a (English)

Working with the Patient Who Has Dementia

☐ The caregiver should eliminate the patient's choices (place only one plate of food and one glass of liquid in front of the patient at a time).

☐ The caregiver should give the patient simple one step instructions (e.g., "Chew your food").

☐ The caregiver should give the patient encouragement to continue eating and drinking.

Therapy Resource 7.31b (Spanish)

Trabajando con el Paciente que Tiene Demencia

☐ El asistente debe eliminar las selecciones del paciente (ponga solo un plato de comida y un vaso de agua a la vez frente al paciente).

☐ El asistente debe darle al paciente instrucciones sencillas (por ejemplo: "Mastique su comida").

☐ El asistente debe animar al paciente para que siga comiendo o tomando.

Therapy Resource 7.32a (English)

The Patient Who Has Had a Stroke

☐ The caregiver should give the patient clear, slow-paced, simple instructions.

☐ The caregiver should model the instructions.

☐ The caregiver should repeat instructions and demonstrations.

☐ The caregiver should give the patient directions on the patient's right side.

☐ The caregiver should give the patient directions on the patient's left side.

☐ The caregiver should present the patient food or liquid where the patient can see.

☐ The caregiver should tap the right or left side of the patient's tray or plate, so the patient can turn to see the rest of the meal.

☐ The caregiver should identify the foods on the patient's tray by telling the patient that the "potatoes are at 12 o'clock and the meat is at 3 o'clock."

☐ The caregiver should turn or reposition the patient's tray if the food or liquid is consumed from only one side of the tray.

Therapy Resource 7.32b (Spanish)

El Paciente Que Ha Tenido Accidente Cerebral

☐ El asistente debe darle al paciente instrucciones lentamente, claras y sencillas.

☐ El asistente debe modelar las instrucciones.

☐ El asistente debe repetir instrucciones y demostraciones.

☐ El asistente debe darle al paciente direcciones en el lado derecho del paciente.

☐ El asistente debe darle al paciente direcciones en el lado izquierdo del paciente.

☐ El asistente debe de presentarle al paciente comida o líquido donde el paciente pueda ver.

☐ El asistente debe dar un golpecito al lado derecho o al lado izquierdo del plato del paciente para que el paciente de vuelta a ver el resto de la comida.

☐ El asistente debe identificar la comida en el plato del paciente por medio de decirle al paciente: "Las papas están a las 12:00 y la carne esta a las 3:00."

☐ El asistente debe voltear o posicionar el plato del paciente, si el paciente solo se ha comido la comida o tomado los líquidos de un lado de su plato.

Therapy Resource 7.33a (English)

The Patient's Oral Care

Before putting food or liquid inside the patient's mouth, the caregiver or another staff member should look inside the mouth. Often, patients with dysphagia have accumulated food or oral secretions inside the mouth that have not been cleaned. The mouth should be cleaned thoroughly for hygiene purposes. Good oral hygiene also provides oral stimulation. This section describes the steps for achieving good oral care.

Cleaning the Mouth

☐ The caregiver should use a moistened Toothette, lemon glycerin swab, or washcloth to clean the mouth. If a washcloth is used, it can be moistened in water containing mouthwash, to freshen as the caregiver cleans the mouth.

☐ The caregiver should start from the outside of the mouth with the washcloth, glycerin swab, or Toothette and go into the mouth.

☐ The caregiver should wipe the patient's lips first. The clinician should remove any flakes or secretions off the patient's lips.

☐ The caregiver should open the patient's lips and wipe the outside of the patient's upper and lower gums.

☐ The caregiver should wipe inside both of the patient's cheeks.

☐ The caregiver should take a toothbrush and toothpaste and brush the outside of the upper and lower teeth. If the patient cannot rinse his or her own mouth, the caregiver should use a wet cloth and wipe the toothpaste off the patient's teeth.

☐ The caregiver should ask the patient to stick out the tongue. Then wipe the tongue using gentle strokes from the back of the tongue to the tip of the tongue. A toothbrush can be used to do this.

☐ The caregiver should ask the patient to open the mouth wide. The caregiver should check the roof of the mouth. The roof of the mouth can be cleaned with a Toothette, lemon glycerin swab, or toothbrush.

☐ The caregiver should wipe the roof of the mouth from the back to the front with gentle strokes.

☐ The caregiver should check to see if there is a mucous plug on the roof of the mouth. This could be dangerous because if the mucous plug is not cleaned out, it could be swallowed by the patient. Once the patient's mouth is cleaned, the caregiver can begin feeding the patient.

Therapy Resource 7.33b (Spanish)

El Cuidado Oral del Paciente

Antes de poner comida o líquido en la boca del paciente, el asistente debe mirar dentro de la boca. Frecuentemente, pacientes con disfagia tienen comida o secreciones que se han acumulado dentro de la boca que no se han limpiado. La boca se debe limpiar completamente por razones de higiene. La buena higiene oral también provee estímulo oral. Esta sección describe los pasos para llevar acabo un buen cuidado oral.

Limpiando la Boca

☐ El asistente debe de usar una esponjita húmeda, un escobillón glicerina de limón o una toallita húmeda para limpiar la boca. Si una toallita es usada, se puede mojar en agua con enjuague bucal, para refrescar mientras que el asistente limpia la boca.

☐ El asistente debe comenzar con la parte afuera de la boca con la toallita, el cotonete glicerina con limón, o la esponjita y después entrar a la boca.

☐ El asistente debe limpiar los labios del paciente primero. El ayudante debe quitar todos los pedazos de piel seca y secreciones de los labios del paciente.

☐ El asistente debe abrir los labios del paciente y limpiar lo de afuera de las encías de arriba y abajo.

☐ El asistente debe limpiar lo de adentro de las dos mejillas del paciente.

☐ El asistente debe tomar un cepillo y pasta de dientes para cepillar lo de afuera de sus dientes de abajo y los de arriba. Si el paciente no se puede enjuagar su propia boca, el asistente debe usar una toallita mojada y limpiar la pasta de los dientes del paciente.

☐ El asistente le debe pedir al paciente que saque la lengua y que limpie la lengua suavemente de atrás hasta la punta de la lengua. Un cepillo de los dientes puede ser usado para hacer esto.

☐ El asistente debe pedirle al paciente que abra la boca ancha. El asistente debe revisar el paladar.

☐ El paladar se puede limpiar con una esponjita, escobillón de glicerina con limón, o un cepillo de dientes.

☐ El asistente debe limpiar el paladar de la boca comenzando por atrás para el frente con pasos suaves.

☐ El asistente debe revisar bien si hay un tapón de mocos en el paladar del paciente. Esto es muy peligroso porque si no se limpia este tapón, el paciente se lo puede tragar. Una vez que este limpia la boca, el asistente puede comenzar a darle comida al paciente.

References

Bartolome, G., & Neumann, S. (1993). Swallowing therapy in patients with neurological disorders causing cricopharyngeal dysfunction. *Dysphagia, 8,* 146–149.

Boshart, C. A. (1998). *Oral-motor analysis and remediation techniques.* Temecula, CA: Speech Dynamics.

Bove, M., Marrison, I., & Eliasson, I. (1998). Thermal oral-pharyngeal stimulation and elicitation of swallowing. *Acta Otolaryngol, 118,* 728–731.

Bryant, M. (1991). Biofeedback in the treatment of a selected dysphagia patient. *Dysphagia, 6,* 140–144.

Buckley, J., Addicks, C., & Maniglia, J. (1976). Feedings patients with dysphagia. *Nursing Forum, 15,* 69–85.

Bulow, M., Olsson, R., & Ekberg, O. (2001). Videomanometric analysis of supraglottic swallow, effortful swallow, and chin tuck in patients with pharyngeal dysfunction. *Dysphagia, 16,* 190–195.

Clark, H. M., Henson, P. H., Barber, W. O., Stierwalt, J. A., & Sherill, M. (2003). Relationships among subjective and objective measures of tongue strength and oral phase I swallowing impairments. *American Journal of Speech-Language Pathology, 12,* 40–50.

Ding, R., Larson, C. W., Logemann, J. A., & Rademaker, A. W. (2002). Surface of electromyographic and electroglottographic studies in normal subjects under two swallow conditions: Normal and during the Mendelsohn Maneuver. *Dysphagia, 17,* 1–12.

Dodds, W. J., Taylor, A. J., Stewart, E. T., Kern, M. K., Logemann, J.A., & Cook, I. J. (1989). Tipper and dipper types of oral swallows. *American Journal of Roentgenology, 153,* 1197–1199.

Donzelli, J., & Brady, S. (2004). The effects of breath-holding on vocal fold adduction: Implications for safe swallowing. *Archives of Otolaryngology–Head & Neck Surgery, 130,* 208–210.

Drake, W., O'Donoghue, S., Bartrum, C., Lindsay, J., & Greenwood, R. (1997). Eating in side-lying position facilitates rehabilitation in neurogenic dysphagia. *Brain Injury, 11,* 137–142.

Easterling, C., Kern, M., Nitscke, T., Grande, B., Daniels, S., Cullen, G. M., et al. (1999). Effect of a novel exercise on swallow function and biomechanics in tube fed cervical dysphagia patients: A preliminary report. *Dysphagia, 14.*

Fujiu, M., & Logemann, J. A. (1996). Effect of tongue-holding maneuver on posterior pharyngeal wall movement during deglutition. *American Journal of Speech-Language Pathology, 5,* 23–30.

Ford, M., Grotz, R., Pomerantz, P., Bruno, R., & Flannery, E. (1974). Dysphagia therapy. *Archives of Physical Medicine and Rehabilitation, 55,* 571.

Gangale, D. (1993). *The source for oral-facial exercises.* East Moline, IL: Linguisystems.

Groher, M. E. (1992). *Dysphagia Diagnosis and Management* (2nd ed.). Stoneham, MA: Butterworth-Heinemann.

Kaatzke-McDonald, M. N., App, M., Post, E., & Davis, P. J. (1996). The effects of cold, touch, and chemical stimulation of the anterior faucial pillar on human swallowing. *Dysphagia, 11,* 198–206.

Kahrilas, P. J., Logemann, J. A., & Gibbons, M. (1992). Food intake by maneuver. An extreme compensation for impaired swallowing. *Dysphagia, 7,* 155–159.

Kahrilas, P. J., Logemann, J. A., Lin, S., & Ergun, G. A. (1992). Pharyngeal clearance during swallow: A combined manometric and videoflouroscopic study. *Gastroenterology, 103,* 128–136.

Larsen, G. (1973). Conservative management for incomplete dysphagia paralytica. *Archives of Physical Medication and Rehabilitation, 54,* 180–185.

Lazarus, C. L., Logemann, J. A., Rademaker, A.W., Kahrilas, P. J., Pajak, T., Lazar, R., et al. (1993). Effects of bolus volume, viscosity, and repeated swallows in nonstroke subjects and stroke patients. *Archives of Physical Medicine and Rehabilitation, 74,* 1066–1070.

Lazarus, C., Logemann, J. A., Song, C. W., Rademaker, A. W., & Kahrilas, P. J. (2002). Effects of voluntary maneuvers on tongue base function for swallowing. *Folia Phoniatrica, 54,* 171–176.

Lazzara, G., Lazarus, C., & Logemann, J. (1986). Impact of thermal stimulation on the triggering of the swallowing reflex. *Dysphagia, 1*, 73–77.

Leonard, R., & Kendall, K. (1997). *Dysphagia assessment and treatment planning: A Team Approach.* San Diego, CA: Singular.

Logemann, J. A. (1993). *Evaluation and treatment of swallowing disorders.* Austin, TX: Pro-Ed.

Logemann, J. A. (1997). Therapy for oropharyngeal swallowing disorders. In A. L. Perlman & K. S. Schulze-Delrieu (Eds.), *Deglutition and its disorders: Anatomy, physiology, clinical diagnosis, and management* (pp. 449–461). San Diego, CA: Singular.

Logemann, J. A. (1998). *Evaluation and treatment of swallowing disorders* (2nd ed.). Austin, TX: Pro-Ed.

Logemann, J. A., & Kahrilas, P. (1990). Relearning to swallow after stroke—application of maneuvers and indirect biofeedback: A case study. *Neurology, 40*, 1136–1138.

Logemann, J. A., Kahrilas, P. J., Cheng, J., Pauloski, B. R., Gibbons, P. J., Rademaker, A. W., et al. (1992). Closure mechanisms of the laryngeal vestibule during swallowing. *American Journal of Physiology, 262*, 6338–6344.

Logemann, J. A., Kahrilas, P. J., Kobara, M., & Vakil, N. (1989). The benefit of head rotation on pharyngoesophageal dysphagia. *Archives of Physical Medicine and Rehabilitation, 70*, 767–771.

Logemann, J. A., Pauloski, B. R., Colangelo, L., Lazarus, C., Fujiu, M., & Kahrilas, P. J. (1995). The Effects of a sour bolus on oropharyngeal swallowing measures in patients with neurogenic dysphagia. *Journal of Speech and Hearing Research, 38*, 556–563.

Logemann, J. A., Pauloski, B. R., Rademaker, A. W., & Colangelo, L. (1997a). Speech and swallowing rehabilitation in head and neck cancer patients. *Oncology, 11*, 651–659.

Logemann, J. A., Pauloski, B. R., Rademaker, A. W., & Colangelo, L. (1997b). Super–supraglottic swallow in irradiated head and neck cancer patients. *Head & Neck, 19*, 535–540.

McCulloch, T. M., Perlman, A. L., Palmer, P. M., & Van Daele, D. J. (1996). Laryngeal activity during swallow, phonation, and the vasalva maneuver: An electromyographic analysis. *Laryngoscope, 106*, 1351–1358.

Martin, B. J. W., Logemann, J. A., Shaker, R., & Dodds, W. J. (1993). Normal laryngeal valving patterns during three breath hold maneuvers: A pilot investigation. *Dysphagia, 8*, 1–20.

Murry, T., & Carrau, R. L. (2006). *Clinical Management of Swallowing Disorders* (2nd ed.). San Deigo, CA: Plural.

O'Sullivan, N., Godfrey, M., van Boldrick, A., & Puntil, J. (1990). *Restorative programs rehab style dysphagia care team approach with acute and long term patients.* Los Angeles: Cottage Square Press.

Perlman, A., & Schultze-Delrieu, K. (1997). *Deglutition and its disorders: Anatomy, physiology, clinical diagnosis and management.* San Diego, CA: Singular.

Perlman, A. (1993). Dysphagia: Evaluation and treatment. The successful treatment of challenging cases. *Clinics in Communication Disorders, 3*, 37–44.

Pounderoux, P., & Kahrilas, P. J. (1995). Deglutitive tongue force modulation by volition, volume, and viscocity in humans. *Gastroenterology, 108*, 1418–1426.

Rademaker, A. W., Logemann, J. A., Pauloski, B. R., Bowman, J., Lazarus, C., Sisson, G., et al. (1993). Recovery of postoperative swallowing in patients undergoing partial laryngectomy. *Head & Neck, 15*, 325–334.

Rasley, A., Logemann, J. A., Kahrilas, P., Rademaker, A. W., Pauloski, B. R., & Dodds, W. J. (1993). Prevention of barium aspiration during videoflouroscopic swallowing studies: Value of change in posture. *AJR American Journal of Roentgenology, 60*, 1005–1009.

Rosenbek, J., Robbins, J., Fishback, B., & Levine, R. (1991). Effects of thermal application on dysphagia after stroke. *Journal of Speech and Hearing Research, 34*, 1257–1268.

Rosenbek, J. C., Robbins, J., Wilford, W., Kirk, G., Schiltz, A., Sowell, T. W., et al. (1998). Comparing treatment intensities of tactile-thermal application. *Dysphagia, 13,* 1–9.

Sciortino, K., Liss, J. M., Case, J. L., Gerritsen, K. G., & Katz, R. C. (2003). Effects of mechanical, cold, gustatory, and combined stimulation to the human anterior faucial arches. *Dysphagia, 18,* 16–26.

Shaker, R., Easterling, C., Kern, M., Nitschke, T., Massey, B., Daniels, S., et al. (2002). Rehabilitation of swallowing by exercise in tube-fed patients with pharyngeal dysphagia secondary to abnormal UES opening. *Gastroenterology, 122,* 1314–1321.

Shaker, R., Kern, M., Bardon, E., Taylor, A., Stewart, E. T., Hoffman, R. G., et al. (1997). Augmentation of deglutitive upper esophageal sphincter opening of the elderly by exercise. *American Journal of Physiology, 272,* 1518–1522.

Shanahan, T. K., Logemann, J. A., Rademaker, A. W., Pauloski, B. R., & Kahrilas, P. J. (1993). Chin down posture effects on aspiration in dysphagic patients. *Archives of Physical Medicine and Rehabilitation, 74,* 736–739.

Silbergleit, A. Waring, W., Sullivan, M., & Maynard, F. (1991). Evaluation, treatment, and follow-up results of post-polio patients with dysphagia. *Otolaryngology–Head and Neck Surgery, 104,* 333–338.

Singh, V. M., Brockbank, J., Frost, R. A., & Tyler, S. (1995). Multi-disciplinary management of dysphagia: The first 100 cases. *The Journal of Laryngology and Otology, 109,* 419–424.

Swigert, N. B. (2000). *The source for dysphagia updated and expanded.* East Moline, IL: Lingui-Sytems.

Welch, M. A., Logemann, J. A., Rademaker, A. W., & Kahrilas, P. J. (1993). Changes in pharyngeal dimensions effected by chin tuck. *Archives of Physical Medicine and Rehabilitation, 74,* 178–181.

English/Spanish Glossary

A

abdomen — estómago

abduct — abducción

ability — habilidad

abnormal — anormal

abscess — absceso, postemilla

absence — falta

absorb — absorber

access — acceso

accident — accidente

accumulate — acumular

accuracy — precisión

achalasia — acalasia

ache — dolor

acid, gastric — ácido gástrico

acidity — acidez

acoustic — acústico

action — acción

activity — actividad

activity, strenuous — actividad fuerte

acute — agudo

Adam's apple — manzana de Adán

adapt — adaptar

add — agregar

address — dirección

adduction — la aducción

adenoids — adenoides

adequate — adecuado, suficiente

adjust — ajustar, adaptar

admission — admisión, ingreso

admit — internar, ingresar

adult — adulto

advance directive — documento que indica de antemano la atención medica deseada en caso de coma y otra incapacidad para expresarse

affect — afecto

affected — afectado

afraid — tener miedo

afternoon — tarde

aftertaste — sabor que queda después de tomar un medicamento o alimento

age — edad

agency — agencia

aggravate — agravar

agile — ágil

aging — envejecimiento

aide — asistente

aide (nurse's) — asistente de enfermería

AIDS (acquired immunodeficiency syndrome) — SIDA

air — aire

airway — via respiratoria aerea

airway closure — cierre de la vía aérea

airway entrance — entrada de la vía aérea

alcohol — alcohol, bebidas alcohólicas

alcoholic — alcohólico

alert — alerta

alignment — alineamiento

all — todo

allergic — alérgico

allergy — alergia

alleviate — aliviar

alternate — alternar

alternating solids and liquids strategy — estrategia de alternar sólidos y líquidos

alveolar ridge — proceso alveolar

alveolus — alveolo

Alzheimer's disease — enfermedad de Alzheimer's

ambulance — ambulancia

ambulatory — ambulatorio

American — americano

amnesia — amnesia

amount — cantidad

amyotrophic lateral sclerosis — esclerosis lateral amiotrofica

anatomy — anatomía

anemia — anemia

anemic — anémico

aneurysm — aneurisma

anger — enojo, coraje

anomaly — anomalía

answer — respuesta

antacid — antiácido

anterior — anterior

Anterior Tongue Click Exercise — ejercicio de clic de lo anterior de la lengua

antibiotic — antibiótico

anticoagulate — anticoagulante

anticonvulsant — anticonvulsivo

antidepressant — antidepresivo

antihistamine — antihistamínico

anti-inflammatory — anti-inflamatorio

antispasmodic — antiespasmódico

anxiety — ansiedad

aphasia — afasia

apnea — apnea del sueño

appetite — apetito

apple — manzana

applesauce — manzana molida

application — aplicación

apply — aplicar

appointment — cita

appropriate — apropiado

apraxia — apraxia

around — alrededor

arouse — despertar

artery — arteria

artery, carotid — arteria carótida

artery, coronary — arteria coronaria

arthritis — artritis

artificial — artificial

artificial sweetener — azúcar artificial

aryepiglottic folds — pliegues ariepigloticos

ascend — ascender

aseptic — aséptico

asleep — dormido

asphyxia — asfixia

aspirate — aspirar

aspiration — aspiración

aspirin — aspirina

assess — evaluar

assist — asistir

assistant, nursing — asistente de enfermería

assure — asegurar

asthma — asma

ataxic — atóxico

ate — comi

atrophy — atrofia

attempt — intento

attend — asistir

attention — atención

atypical — atípico

audiogram — audiograma

audiologist — audiologo

audiology — audiologia

audiometer — audiometro

audition — audición

auditory — auditivo

auditory tube — conducto auditivo

aunt — tía

avoid — evitar

awake — despierto

awareness — conocimiento

B

Back Tongue Push-up Exercise — ejercicio de levantar la parte posterior de la lengua

Back Tongue Tickle — cosquilleo de la lengua posterior

backache — dolor de espalda

backward — hacia atrás

bacterial — bacteriano

bad — malo

bake — hornear

balance — balance, equilibrio

bandage — vendaje

barium — bario

barrier — barrera

basal ganglia — ganglios básales

basic — básico

bath — baño

bed — cama

bedding — ropa de cama

bedridden — confinado en cama, encamado

bedside — lado de la cama

bedsore — llaga, ulcera

beginning — comienzo, principio

behavior — conducta, comportamiento

behind — trasero

Bell's palsy — parálisis facial de Bell

bellyache — cólico, dolor de barriga

bend — doblar, inclinar

benefit — beneficio

better — mejor

big — grande

Big Smile Exercise — ejercicio de sonrisa grande

big yawn — bostezo grande

Big Yawn Exercise — ejercicio de bostezeo

bilateral — bilateral

bile — bilis

bilingual — bilingüe

bill — cuenta, cobro

binge — juerga

biofeedback — bioretroalimentación

biopsy — biopsia

bite — morder/mordida/bocado

bitter — agrio, amargo

Bitter Press — presión amarga

bland — sin sabor fuerte

blanket — cobija

bleed — sangrar

blind — ciego

blink — parpadeo

blister — ampolla

bloated — hinchado

blocked — tapado

blood — sangre

blood pressure — presión arterial

blood thinner — anticoagulante

bloody nose — sangrando por la nariz

blow one's nose — sonarse la nariz

blurred vision — vista nublada

blurry — empando, borroso

bolus — bolo

Bolus Control Exercises — ejercicios para control del bolo

Bolus Exercises — ejercicios para el bolo

bone — hueso

bowel movement — evacuación de heces fecales

brace — aparato corrector

brain — cerebro

brainstem — tronco cerebral

breakfast — desayuno

breath — aliento, rcspiro, respiracion

breathe — respirar

breathing difficulty — dificultad para respirar

bronchitis — bronquitis

bronchopneumonia — bronconeumonía

bronchus — bronquio

broth — caldo

bruise — contusion

brush — cepillo

buccal cavity — cavidad bucal

buildup — deposito, acumulación

burn — quemada, quemar, arder

burning — ardiente, quemante

burp — erutar

C

caffeine — cafeína

calcium — calcio

calm — tranquilo

calorie — caloría

canal, auditory — canal auditivo

cancel — cancelar

cancer — cáncer

candy — dulce

cane — bastón

canker sore — pequeña úlcera en la boca

carbonated — carbónico

cardiac — cardiaco

care — cuidado, atención

caregiver — cuidador

carotid — carótida

cartilage — cartílago

cataract — catarata

catheter — catéter

cause — causar

center — centro

cereal — cereal

cerebellum — cerebelo

cerebral palsy — parálisis cerebral

cerebrum — cerebro

cerumen — cera del oído

chair — silla

change — cambio

Chapstick — pomada de labios

check — revisar

cheek — mejilla

Cheek Puff Exercise — ejercicio de soplo de mejilla

Cheek Push Strategy — estrategia del empujon de la mejilla

Cheek Push-up Exercise — ejercicio de levantar la mejilla

chemotherapy — quimioterapia

chest x-ray (film) — radiografía del tórax

chew — masticar

chewing gum — chicle

Chewing Gum or Licorice Exercise — ejercicio de chicle o regaliz

chill — escalofrió

chin — barba, barbilla

Chin Tuck Strategy — estrategia de barbilla hacia abajo

choke — ahogarse

cholesterol — colesterol

chorea, Huntington's — corea de Huntington

chronic — crónico

chromosome — cromosoma

cigarette — cigarro

Circular Dry Gauze Chew Exercise — ejercicio de masticar la gasa seca en movimiento circular

circulation — circulación

cirrhosis — cirrosis

clammy — pegajoso y frío

clean — limpio

clear — aclarar, limpiar

clear the throat — aclarar la garganta

cleft palate — paladar hendido

clinic — clínica

clinician — medico clínico

clockwise — sentido de las agujas del reloj

close — cerrar

Close/Open Lip Exercise — ejercicio de abrir y cerrar los labios

clot — coagular

clothes — ropa

coat — abrigo

coated — cubierto

cochlea — coclea

cognition — cognición

cohesive — cohesivo/cohesiva

Coke — coca

cold — frío

Cold Bolus Strategy — estrategia de bolo frío

Cold Inner Cheek Rub — rozar frío del interior de la mejilla

Cold Lip Rub — rozar frío el labio

cold sore — úlcera en los labios

collapse — colapso [noun]

collapse, lung — colapso pulmonar

collect — recoger

colors — colores

comatose — comatoso

comb — peine

comfortable — cómodo

communicate — comunicar

communication — comunicación

compatible — compatible

compensate — compensar

complain — quejarse

complaint — queja

complement — complemento

complete — completo

completely — completamente

complication — complicación

concentrate — concentrar

concentration — concentración

concussion — concusión

condition — condición

confidential — confidencial

confused — confundido/confundida

congestion — congestión

consciousness, lose — perder el conocimiento

consent — consentimiento, permiso

consistency — consistencia

consistency of food — consistencia de la comida

constrict — apretar, compresar

consult — consultar

consumption — consumo

contact — contacto

contagious — contagioso

continue — continuar

contract — contraer [verb]; contrato [noun]

contraction — contracción

control — controlar

convalescent — convaleciente

convulsion — convulsión

cooperate — cooperar

cooperative — cooperativo

corner — esquina

correct — correcto

cortex — corteza

cough — tos

count — recuento

cover — cubrir

cranberry — arandano

cranial — craneal

cranial nerves — nervios craneales

craving — antojos

cricoid cartilage — cartílago cricoide

cricopharyngeal sphincter — esfinter cricofaringeal

cried — lloro

critical — crítico

crooked — torcido

crush — macular, aplastar

cry — llanto

culture — cultura

cup — taza

cushion — cojín

cut — cortar

cyst — quiste o bolsa de pus

cystic fibrosis — fibrosis quistita

D

Dad — papá

dairy product — producto de leche

dangerous — peligroso

date — cita

daughter — hija

daughter-in-law — nuera

day — día

day, every — todos los días

days of the week — días de la semana

dead — muerte

deaf — sordo/sorda

debilitating — debilitante

deceased — difunto

decision — decisión

decongestant — descongestionante

decrease — disminuir

deep — hondo, profundo

deep breath — respiración profunda

defense mechanism — mecanismo de defensa

deficiency — deficiencia

deficit — déficit

degenerative — degenerativo

degenerative disease — enfermedad degenerativa

dehydration — deshidratado/deshidrata

delayed — retrasado

delirious — delirante

dementia — demencia

demonstrate — demonstrar

denial — negación

dentist — dentista

denture, partial — dentadura parcial

dentures — dentadura postiza

dependent — dependiente

depletion — agotamiento

depressed — deprimido

depression — depresion

depressor, tongue — depresor de lengua

describe — describir

desensitize — desensibilizar

desire — desear

dessert — postre

detect — detectar

deteriorate — empeorarse

determine — determinar

device — aparato

diabetes — diabetes

diabetic — diabético

diagnose — diagnosticar

diagnosis — diagnóstico

dialysis — diálisis

diaphragm — diafragma

diarrhea — diarrea

die — morir

diet — dieta

diet change — el cambio de dieta

dietitian — especialista en dietética

difficult — difícil

difficulty breathing — dificultad para respirar

difficulty swallowing — dificultad para tragar

digest — digerir

digestion — digestión

dinner — cena

direction — dirección

dirty — sucio

dirty (to get) — ensuciar

discharge (secretion) — secreción

discharge from hospital — dar de alta

discomfort — molestia

disease — enfermedad

disinfect — desinfectar

disinfectant — desinfectante

disorder — desorden

disoriented — desorientado/desorientada

disposable — desechable

dissolve — disolver

distraction — distracción

distress — aflicción

diuretic — diurético

dizziness — mareo

dizzy — mareado

do — hacer

doctor — médico

dominant — dominante

dopamine — dopamina

dose — dosis

downward — hacia abajo

drainage — drenaje

drink — bebida

drip — gotear

drool — babear [verb]; baba [noun]

drowsy — somnoliento

drug — droga

drugstore — farmacia

dry — seco

Dry Gargle Exercise — ejercicio de gárgara seca

dry mouth — boca seca

dryness — sequedad

dull pain — dolor calmado

Dump and Swallow Strategy — estrategia de descargar y tragar

Dump and Swallow with the Supraglottic Swallow Strategy — estrategia de descargar y tragar con supraglottic

duration — duración

during — durante

dye — colorante

dysphagia — disfagia

E

ear — oido

ear wax — cerilla

earache — dolor de oído

easily — facilidad

eat — comer

educate — educar

effective — efectivo

efficient — eficiente

effort — esfuerzo

Effortful Swallow Exercise/Strategy — ejercicio/estrategia de trago con esfuerzo

elderly — anciano

elevate — elevar

elevation — elevación

embolism — embolia

embolism (pulmonary) — embolia pulmonar

emergency — emergencia

emesis basin — escupidera

emotion — emoción

emotional — emocional

emphasis — énfasis

empty — vació

Empty Mouth Strategy — estrategia de la boca vacía

encephalitis — encefalitis

endoscope — endoscopio

endoscopy — endoscopia

energetic — enérgico

energy — energía

enlarge — aumentar

ENT (ear-nose-throat specialist) — especialista de oídos, nariz, y garganta

enter — entrar

entrance — entrada

environment — ambiente

epiglottis — epiglotis

epilepsy — epilepsia

episode — episodio

equilibrium — equilibrio

esophageal phase — fase esofagea

esophageal reflux — reflujo esófageal

esophagitis — esofagitis

esophagus — esófago

ethical — ético

eustachian tube — trompa de eustaquio

evaluate — evaluar

evaluation — evaluación

eventually — con el tiempo

examination — examinación

examine — examinar

excess — exceso

excessive — excesivo/excesiva

exercise — ejercicio

exercise tolerance — tolerancia al ejercicio

exhale — exhalar

expect — esperar

expel — expulsar

expire — fallecer, expirar

explain — explicar

exposure — exposición

extensive — extenso

eye — ojo

F

face — cara

face down — boca abajo

face up — boca arriba

faint — mareado

faith healer — curandero

faith healing — curanderismo

fall — caer [verb]; caída [noun]

fall out — salga

fall out of the mouth — caerse de la boca

Falsetto/Pitch Exercise — ejercicio de nivel falsete

family — familia

fast — rápido/rápida

faster — más rápido

fasting — en ayunas

fatal — fatal, mortal

father — padre

father-in-law — suegro

fatigue — fatiga

faucial arches — arcos faucales

faucial pillars — pilares faucales

fear — miedo

feed — alimentar, dar de comer

feel — sentir

feeling — sensación

female — femenino/a [sex]; hembra [animal]

fever — fiebre

fever blister — ampolla de fiebre en los labios

few — pocos

fibrosis — fibrosis

field worker — campesino

fill — llenar

finding — descubrimiento

finger — dedo

finish — acabar

fire — fuego

firm — firme

first — primero

fistula — fístula

fit — ajustar

fix — reparar

flaccid — flaccido

flat — plano

flatulence — flatulencia

flavor — sabor

flexible — flexible

flow — flujo

flu — influenza

fluid — líquidos

fluoroscopy — fluoroscopia

focus — foco

focusing — enfocar

follow — seguir

follow-up, medical — atención médica subsecuente

food — comida

Food Hold Strategy — estrategia de sostener la comida

force — fuerza

forcefully — forzosamente

forehead — frente

forget — olvidar

fork — tenedor

form — formar

formation — formación

formula — formula

forward — hacia adelante

fragile — fragil

frail — fragil, debil

freeze — congelar

frequently — frecuentemente

fresh — fresco

friend — amigo/amiga

front — enfrente

frown — fruncir el ceno

frozen — congelado/congelada

full — lleno

function — funcionar [verb]; función [noun]

fuse — fusionar

G

gag reflex — reflejo de atragantarse

gain weight — aumentar de peso

gallbladder — vesícula biliar

gallstone — calculo biliar

ganglion — ganglio

gangrene — gangrena

gargle — harcer gárgaras

gargling — gárgara

gas, to have — tener gas

gasp — hacer esfuerzos para respirar

gastrectomy — gastrectomía

gastroenterologist — gastroenterólogo

gastrostomy — gastronomía

gauze — gasa

generic — genérico

gentle — suave

gently — suavemente

geriactrics — geriatría

geriatric — geriatric

gesture — gesto

girl — niña, muchacha

girlfriend — novia

give — dar

gland — glándula

gland, salivary — glándula salival

glass — vaso

glasses — lentes

glaucoma — glaucoma

glossitis — glositis

glossopharyngeal nerve — nervio glosofaringeo

glottis — glotis

glove — guante

glucose — glucosa

goal — meta

good — bueno

gown — bata

gradually — poco a poco, gradualmente

grandchild — nieto/nieta

granddaughter — nieta

grandfather — abuelo

grandmother — abuela

grasp — agarrar

grease — grasa

greasy — grasoso

green — verde

grieve — afligirse

grimace — hacer muecas

grind — moler

groan — gemido

guardian — guardian

guide — guía

guidelines — las directrices

gum — encía

gurgle — gorgotear

H

habit [noun] — hábito

habit [verb] — habituar

habit-forming — que crea hábito

hair — pelo

half — medio

halitosis — mal aliento

hand — mano

handkerchief — pañuelo

handling — manejo

handwriting — escritura

happy — feliz, contento

hard — duro

hard palate — paladar duro

harm —dañar [verb]; daño [noun]

hazard — peligro

head — cabeza

Head Forward Position Strategy — estrategia posición con la cabeza hacia abajo

Head Tilt Strategy — estrategia de inclinar la cabeza

Head Turn Exercise/Strategy — ejercicio/estrategia de voltear la cabeza

Head Turn with Chin Down Strategy — estrategia de barbilla hacia abajo con la cabeza volteada

headache — dolor de cabeza

health — salud

healthy — sano

hear — oír

heart — corazón

heartburn — agruras

Heimlich maneuver — maniobra de Heimlich

help — ayudar

hemiplegia — hemiplejia

hemisphere — hemisferio

hemorrhage — hemorragia

heparin — heparina

hepatitis — hepatitis

hernia — hernia

hernia (hiatal) — hernia hiatal

hiccup — hipo

high — alto

high blood pressure — alta presión de sangre

high-pitched — de tono alto

high-risk — alto riesgo

history (medical) — historia clínica

hoarse — ronco/ronca

hoarseness — ronquera

hold — detener, retener

hold one's breath — detener la respiración

hold one's nose — detener la nariz

home — casa

homemade — hecho en casa

hormone — hormona

hospice — asilo para pacientes con enfermedades terminales

hospital — hospital

hot (to taste) — picante

hot (to touch) — caliente, calor

hour — hora

hungry, to be — tener hambre

hurt — doler

husband — esposo

hydrate — hidratar

hygiene, oral — aseo oral

hyoid bone — hueso hoides

hypersensitive — hipersensible

hypertension — hipertensió

hyperventilate — respirar demasiado rápido, hiperventilado

hypothalamus — hipotálamo

hypothyroid— hipotiroidismo

hyrocephaly — hidrocefalia

I

ice — hielo

ice chips — pedacitos de hielo

ice cream — helado

ice pack — bolsa de hielo

Iced Cheek Technique — técnica de mejilla helada

identify — identificar

ill — enfermo

imbalance — desequilibrio

immediate — inmediato/inmediata

immediately — inmediatamente

immunization — inmunización

impair — dañar

impairment — daño

important — importante

improve — mejorar

impulsive — impulsivo

in — dentro

incisor — diente incisivo

incomplete — incompleto

increase — aumentar

independent — independiente

indication — indicación

indigestion — indigestión

infarct — infarto

infection — infección

inflammation — inflamación

ingest — ingerir

inhale — inhalar

initial — inicial

inner — interno

inside — dentro

instruction — instrucción

insulin — insulina

insurance — seguro

intact — intacto

intensive — intensivo

interpret — interpretar

intervention — intervención

intestine — intestino

intracranial — intracraneal

intubate — intubar

invasive — invasor

involuntary — involuntario

irregular — irregular

irritable — irritable

itch — picazón

J

jaundice — ictericia

jaw, lower — maxilar inferior

jaw, upper — maxilar superior

jawbone — mandíbula, quijada

jejunal tube — tubo de yeyuno

jejunum — yeyuno

job — trabajo

join — ligar, juntar

joint — articulación

juice — jugo

K

/k/ Tongue Production Exercise — ejercicio de producción de lengua con sonido /k/

ketoacidosis — cetoacidosis

kidney — riñón

kidney disease — enfermedad de los riñones

kidney failure — insuficiencia renal

kidney stone — calculo renal

kind — amable, cosiderado

kind (type) — clase

kiss — besar [verb]; beso [noun]

knees — rodillas

knife-like (pain) — punzante

knives — cuchillos

L

labial — labial

labial seal — sello de labios

labyrinth — laberinto

laceration — laceración

lack — deficiencia, falta

lactose — lactosa

lactose intolerant — intolerancia a la lactosa

lamp — lámpara

language — lenguaje

lard — manteca

large — grande

Large Bolus Strategy — estrategia de bolo grande

laryngeal — laríngeo

laryngectomy — laringectomía

laryngitis — laringitis

laryngoscopy — laringoscopia

larynx — laringe

last — último

lateral — lateral

Lateral Chew Exercise — ejercicio de masticar lateral

Lateral Lick Exercise — ejercicio de lamido lateral

Lateral Tongue Push Exercise — ejercicio de empujón de los lados de la lengua

Lateral Tongue Push Exercise — ejercicio de los lados de la lengua

lateralization — la lateralización

laugh — risa

laxative — laxante

lean — inclinar

lean backward — inclinese hacia atras

lean forward — inclinese hacia adelante

lean to your side — inclinese a su lado

left — izquierdo/izquierda

left-handed — zurdo

legs — piernas

lemon — limón

lemon glycerin swab — aplicador de limón y glicerina

lesion — lesión

lethargic — letárgico

leukemia — leucemia

lick — lamer; lama

lie down — acostarse

life support — se refiere a equipos y métodos para sostener funciones vitales como la respiración

life-threatening — que amenaza la vida

lift — levantar

light — luz

lightheaded, to feel — tener mareo

limit — limitar [verb]; límite [noun]

lingual — lingual

lining — revestimiento

lip — labio

lip, lower — labio inferior

lip, upper — labio superior

Lip Rub Exercise — ejercicio de rozar los labios

lip seal — sello de labios

Lip Squeeze Exercise — ejercicio de apretar los labios

liquid — líquido

liquid barium — bario líquido

lisp — ceceo

listen — escuchar

little — pequeño

little bit — poco

liver — hígado

liver disease — enfermedad del hígado

liver failure — insuficiencia hepática

lobe — lóbulo

lockjaw — mandíbula cerrada

long-term — a largo plazo

look — mirar

lose — perder

lose weight — perder peso

loss — pérdida

loss of balance — pérdida del equilibrio

loss of consciousness — pérdida del conocimiento

loss of hearing — pérdida de la audición

loss of memory — pérdida de la memoria

loss of sensation — pérdida de la sensibilidad

loud — fuerte

love — amor

loved one — ser amado

low — bajo

lower — abajo

Lower Lip Push-up Exercise — ejercicio de levantar el labio inferior

low-pitched — tono grave

lozenge — trocisco de pastilla para chupar

lukewarm — templado/templada, tibio

lunch — comida

lung/lungs — pulmón/pulmoncs

Lying Down on the Side Strategy — estrategia de tendido en el lado

lymph node — ganglio

lymphoma — linfoma

M

mad — enojado

magnetic resonance imaging (MRI) — imágenes por resonancia magnética

maintain — mantener

malaria — paludismo, malaria

male — masculino, varon

malignant — maligno

malnourished — desnutrido

malnutrition — desnutrición

man — hombre

manage — manejar, dirigir

mandible — mandíbula

maneuver — maniobra

manipulate — manipular

manubrium — manubrio

many — muchos

many times — muchas veces

mash — machacar

mask — en máscara

mass — masa

massage — masaje

massive — masivo

mastoid — mastoideo

mastoid process — apófisis mastoidea

material — material

matter, gray — substancia gris

matter, white — substancia blanca

mattress — colchón

maxilla — maxilar

maxillofacial — maxilofacial

maximum — máximo

may — tal vez

meal — comida

measure — medida

meat — carne

mechanism — mecanismo

medial — intermedio

medical — médico

medications — medicamentos

medicine — medicina

medico history — historial médico

medulla — bulbo raquídeo

membrane — membrana

membrane (mucous) — membrana mucosa

membrane (tympanic) — membrana timpánica

memory — memoria

memory (long-term) — memoria remota

memory (short-term) — memoria reciente

memory loss — perdida de la memoria

men — hombres

Mendelsohn maneuver — maniobra Mendelsohn

Mendelsohn Maneuver Exercise — ejercicio de maniobra de Mendelsohn

meninges — meninges

meningitis — meningitis

metabolic — metabólico

metabolism — metabolismo

meter — metro

method — método

Mexican — mexicano/mexicana

midbrain — cerebro medio

middle — medio

Middle Tongue Pop Exercise — ejercicio de explosión con el medio de la lengua

Middle Tongue Push Exercise — ejercicio de empujón con el medio de la lengua

Midline Food Position Strategy — estrategia de posición de comida en medio de la lengua

mild — leve

milk — leche

Milk of Magnesia — leche de magnesia

milkshake — licuado, batido de leche

milligram — miligramo

milliliter — mililitro

millimeter — milímetro

minimum — mínimo

minute — minuto

mirror — espejo

mirror, laryngeal — espejo laríngeo

miss — faltar

mix — mezclar

mixture — mezcla

moan — gemido [noun]; gemir [verb]

mobile — móvil

mobility — movilidad

model — modelar

moderate — moderado

moderation — moderación

modification — modificación

modified barium swallow study — estudio de la deglución de bario modificado

Modified Tongue Anchor Exercise — ejercicio modificado de anclar la lengua

Modified Tongue Sqeeze Strategy — estrategia de apretón de lengua modificado

Modified Tongue Tip Sweep Exercise — ejercicio de barrer con la punta de la lengua modificado

modify — modificar

moist — humedo

moisten — humedecer, mojar un poco

Mom — mamá

monitor — monitor

morning — de la mañana

mother — madre

mother-in-law — suegra

motivation — motivación

mouth — boca

mouth (roof of) — paladar

Mouth Rinse Strategy — estrategia de enjuago de la boca

mouthful — bocado

mouthwash — enjuage bucal

move — mover

movement — movimiento

much — mucho

mucous — mucoso

mucous membrane — membrana mucosa

multiple sclerosis — esclerosis múltiple

Multiple Swallow Strategy — estrategia de trago múltiple

mumps — paperas

murmur — soplo

muscle — músculo

muscle weakness — debilidad muscular

muscular dystrophy — distrofia muscular progresiva

myasthenia gravis — miastenia grave

myelin — mielina

myocardial infarction — infarto de miocardio

N

name — nombre

name, first — primer nombre

name, last — apellido

nap — siesta

napkin — servilleta

narrow — estrecho

nasal — nasal

nasal (resonance) — gangoso

nasal cavity — cavidad nasal

nasal passage — conducto nasal

nasogastric — nasogástrico

nasogastric tube — tubo nasogástrico

nasopharynx — nasofaringe

nausea — náusea

nauseated, to be — tener náusea

nauseous — que tiene náusea

necessary — necesario

neck — cuello

nectar — néctar

neglect — negligencia

nephew — sobrino

nerve — nervio

nerve, cranial — nervio craneal

nerve, phrenic — nervio frenico

nerve, recurrent laryngeal — nervio laríngeo recurrente

nerve, sensory — nervio sensitivo

nerve, trigeminal — nervio trigémino

nerve, vagus — nervio vago

nervous — nervioso

neural — neural

neurogenic — neurogènico

neurological — neurológico

neurologist — neurólogo/neuróloga

neurology — neurología

neurosurgeon — neurocirujano/ neurocirujana

next — luego, otro

niece — sobrina

night — noche

night, last — anoche

nodule — nódulo

noise — ruido

noninvasive — invasor

noon — mediodía

normal — normal

nose — nariz

nothing by mouth (NPO) — nada por la boca

notice — notar

nourishment — nutrición

numb — dormido

numbness — adormecimiento

nurse — enfermera

nutrition — nutrición

nutritionist — especialista en nutrición

O

obese — obeso

obesity — obesidad

object — objeto

observe — observar, observe

obstruct — obstruir

obstruction — obstrucción

occipital — occipital

occlusion — oclusión

occupation — ocupación

occur — ocurrir

odor — olor

office — oficina

often — seguido

"Oh" Lips Exercise — ejercicio de "O" de labios

ointment — pomada

one-fourth — un cuartro

one-half— un medio/una media

one-third — un tercio

onset — comienzo, principio

open — abrir

open your mouth — abra la boca

operate — operar

operation — operación

ophthalmologist — oftalmólogo

opinion — opinion

optometrist — optometrista

oral — oral

oral cavity — cavidad oral

oral examination — examen oral

oral exercise — ejercicios de la boca

oral phase — la fase oral

oral preparatory phase — la fase oral preparatoria

order — ordenar

organ — órgano

oropharnx — orofaringe

oropharyngeal area — área oro faríngea

orthodontist — orthodoncista

osteoarthritis — osteoartritis

otitis — otitis

otitis media — otitis media

otolaryngologist — otorrinolaringólogo/otorrinolaringóloga

otoscope — otoscopia

ouch! — ¡ay!

ounce — onza

out — afuera

Out/In Tongue Exercise — ejercicio de la lengua para fuera y para adentro

outcome — resultado

outer — externo

outpatient — paciente externo

overexert — agotar

over-the-counter — que no requiere receta medica

oxigeno — oxígeno

oxygen tank — tanque de oxígeno

P

page (overhead) — llamada por bocina

page (from pager/beeper) — llamada por el biper

pager — biper

pain — dolor

painful — doloroso

palatable — de sabor aceptable

palate — paladar

palate, cleft — paladar hendido

palate, hard — paladar duro

palate, soft — paladar blando

palpate — palpar

palsy — parálisis

palsy (Bell's) — parálisis de Bell

pancreas — páncreas

panic — pánico

papilla — papila

paralyze — paralizar

parent — padre

paresis — paresia

parietal — parietal

part — parte

partial — parcial

pass — pasar [verb]; paso [noun]

passive — pasivo

paste — pasta

patience — paciencia

patient — paciente

peel — pelar

penetration — penetración

peptic ulcer — úlcera péptica

perception — percepción

performance — rendimiento

peripheral — periférico

peristalsis — perístasis

peristaltic waves — ondas peristálticas

peritoneum — peritoneo

permanent — permanente

permission — permiso

permit — permitir; permita

persist — persistir

pharmacist — farmacéutico

pharmacy — farmacia

pharyngeal phase — fase faríngea

pharyngitis — faringitis

pharynx — faringe

phase — fase

phlebotomist — flebotomista

phlegm — flema

phrase — frase

phrenic — frenico

physician — médico

piece — pedazo

piercing — penetrante

pill (capsule) — cápsula

pill (solid) — píldora, pastilla, tableta

pillow — almohada

pint — pinta

pitcher — jarra

pituitary — pituitario

plastic — plástico

plate — plato

please — por favor

pneumonia — pulmonía

pneumonia, aspiration — pulmonía por aspiración

podiatrist — podiatra

point — apuntar [verb]; apunte [noun]

polyp — pólipo

pons — puente

portable — portátil

portion — porción

position — posición

posterior — posterior

Posterior Food Position Strategy — estrategia de posición de la comida en la parte posterior

postnasal — postnasal

postnasal drip — secreción nasal posterior

postpone — aplazar, posponer

posture — postura

potential — potencial

pound — libra

powder — polvo

powdered — en polvo

precaution — precaución

precise — preciso

premature spillage — derrame prematuro

preparation — preparación

prepare — preparar

presbycusis — presbiacusia

presentation — presentación

press — aplanar

pressure — presión

pretend — pretender

prevalence — prevalencia

prevent — prevenir

prevention — prevención

previous — previo

primary — primario

privacy — privacidad

probably — probablemente

problem — problema

procedure — procedimiento

process — apófisis

produce — producir

professional — profesional

prognosis — pronóstico

program — programa

progress — progreso

propel — propulsar

proprioceptive — propioceptivo

prosthesis — prótesis

prosthetic — protésica

protect — proteger

provide — suministrar, proporcionar

psychiatrist — psiquiatra

psychologist — psicólogo

Pucker and Smile Exercise — ejercicio de fruncir y sonreír

Puerto Rican — puertorriqueño

puff — inflar, infle

pull — estirar

pull back — tire hacia atrás

Pulling Exercise — ejercicio de tirón

pulse — pulso

pureed — puré

push — empujar

Pushing Exercise — ejercicio de empujón

put — poner

pyriform sinus — seno piriforme

Q

quality — calidad

quality of life — calidad de vida

quart — cuarto

queasy — con un poco de nausea

question — pregunta

questionnaire — cuestionario

questions — preguntas

quiet — quieto, silencio

quit — dejar de, parar

R

radiation — radiación

radiologist — radiólogo

radiology — radiología

raise — levantar, elevar

range of motion — campo de movimiento

rare — raro

rash — erupción

rate — velocidad

raw — crudo

reaction — reacción

read — leer

recently — recientemente

recommend — recomendar

recommendation — recomendación

recover — recuperar

recovery — recuperación

recuperate — recuperarse

recurrence — recurrencia

reduce — reducir

Reduced Bolus Size Strategy — estrategia de bolo reducido en tamaño

reflex — reflejo

reflex, gag — reflejo nauseoso

reflux — reflujo

reflux, esophageal — reflujo esofágico

regain — recuperar

regular — regular

regurgitate — regurgitar

regurgitation — regurgitación

rehabilitation — rehabilitación

reinforce — reforzar

relax — relajar

release — alojar

remember — recordar, acordarse

remove — extraer, sacar, quitar, remover

renal — renal

renal failure — insuficiencia renal

repeat — repetir

report — reportar

residue — residuo

resistance — resistencia

respiration — respiración

respirator — respirador

respiratory distress — dificultades respiratorias

respiratory failure — insuficiencia respiratoria

respond — responder

response — respuesta

rest [verb] — descansar

rest (remainder) — resto

restraints — sujetadores

restroom — baño

resuscitate — resucitar

rhythm — ritmo

rib — costilla

rib cage — caja torácica

rice pudding — atole de arroz

right — derecha

right (moral) — derecho

rigid — rígido

rinse — enjuagar

risk — riesgo

risk factor — factor de riesgo

rolling motion — movimiento rodante

roof of mouth — paladar

room — cuarto, habitación

rough — áspero

round — redondo

rounds — redondear

rub — rozar, frotar, tallar

runny — líquido, de consistencia licuada

S

sad — triste

safe — seguro

safety — seguridad

saliva — saliva

salt — sal

salty — salado

say — decir, diga

scan, CT — tomografía axial computarizada

scared to be — tener miedo

screen — examen de detección

screening — detección

second — segundo

secrete — secretar

secretion — secreción

secretions — secreciones

seizure — ataque convulsivo

senior citizen — persona anciana

sensation — sensación

sense — sentido

sensitive — sensible

sensory — sensorial

sensory (nerve) — sensitivo

sensory (perception) — sensorio

sepsis — sepsis

septic — séptico

serious — serio

service — servicio

serving — porción

severe — severo

severity — gravedad

sharp — agudo/aguda

sheet — sabana

shirt — camisa

shoe — zapato

shooting (pain) — punzante

shortness of breath — sensación de ahogo

short-term — corto plazo

show — enseñar

shy — tímido

sibling — hermano/hermana

sick — enfermo

side — lado

side effect — efecto colateral

Side Pucker Exercise — ejercicio de fruncir el lado

siderail — barandal, baranda

Side Tongue Hold Exercise — ejercicio de agarrar el lado de la lengua

Side-to-Side Tongue Wag Exercise — ejercicio de maneo de lengua de lado a lado

sign — signo, gesto

signature — firma

silent aspiration — aspiración silenciosa

sink — lavamanos

sip — sorber [verb]; sorbo [noun]

sister — hermana

sister-in-law — cuñada

sit — sientese

sit up — sientese derecho

skill — destreza, habilidad

skull — cráneo

sleep — sueño

slow — lento/lenta

slowly — lentamente

slur (one's words), to — hablar con la lengua pesada

Small Bolus Strategy — estrategia de bolo pequeño

smell — olor

smell bad — oler mal

smile — sonreír [verb]; sonrisa [noun]

smoke — fumar

smoker — fumador

snack — bocadillo

soak — remojar

social service — servicio social

social worker — trabajador social/ trabajadora social

soda — soda

soft — blando

soft — suave

soft drink — refresco

Soft Lip Press — presión suave al labio

solid — sólido

solid food — comida sólida

son — hijo

son-in-law — yerno

sore — adolorido, llaga, úlcera

sore throat — dolor de garganta

sound — sonido

soup — sopa, caldo

sour — agrio/agria

Sour Bolus Strategy — estrategia de bolo amargo

spastic — espástico

speak — hablar

specialist — especialista

specific — específico

speech — habla

speech-language pathologist, female — la patóloga de habla y lenguaje

speech-language pathologist, male — el patólogo de habla y lenguaje

speed — velocidad

spicy — picante

spill — derramar, tirar

spinal cord — médula espinal

spit— escupir [verb]; saliva [noun]

spleen — bazo

spontaneous — espontáneo

spoon — cuchara

Spoon Press Strategy — estrategia de apretón con cuchara

spoonful — cucharada

sputum — esputo, flema

squeeze — apretar

stabilize — estabilizar

stable — estable

stage — etapa

stand — levantarse, levantese

starch — almidón

start — comenzar

status — estado

stay — quedar

stenosis — estenosis

stepbrother — hermanastro

stepdaughter — hijastra

stepfather — padrastro

stepmother — madrastra

stepsister —hermanastra

stick — pegar, secar

stick out your tongue — saque la lengua

stiff— rígido

stiffness — rigidez

stimulate — estimular

stimulus — estímulo

stoma, tracheal — abertura de la tráquea

stomach — estómago

stomachache — dolor de estómago

stop — parar

straight — derecho

strategy — estrategia

straw — popote

strength — fuerza, vigor

strengthen — esforzar

stress — tensión

stretch — estirar

stricture — estenosis

strike [verb] — derramar

stroke (i.e., CVA) — derrame sonrisa cerebral

strong — fuerte

Strong Hold Food Strategy — estrategia de sostener fuerte la comida

stuck — atorar

stutter — tartamudear

subacute — subagudo

subdural — subdural

substitute — substituto

suck — chupar

Suck Swallow Exercise — ejercicio de trago de chupar

suction — succión

suddenly — de repente

sufficient — suficiente

sugar — azúcar

sugarless — sin azúcar

Super-Supraglottic Swallow Exercise/ Strategy — ejercicio/estrategia de trago super-supraglottic

supplement — suplemento

Supraglottic Swallow Exercise/Strategy — ejercicio/estrategia de trago supraglottic

sure — seguro, cierto

surgeon — cirujano/cirujana

surgery — cirugía

sustain — sostener, sostenga

Swab Swipe Exercise — limpiar con aplicador

swallow [verb] — tragar

swallow, delayed — deglución retrasada

swallow, incomplete — deglución incompleta

swallow, please — trague, por favor

swallow, super-supraglottic — deglución super-supraglotica

swallowing reflex — reflejo de deglución

sweet — dulce

sweets — dulces

swelling — hinchazón

swollen — hinchado

sympathetic, to be — tener compasión

sympathetic nervous system — sistema nervioso simpático

symptom — síntoma

syndrome — síndrome

syndrome, acquired immunodeficiency (AIDS) — síndrome de immunodeficiencia adquirida (SIDA)

syndrome, Guillain-Barré — síndrome de Guillain-Barré

syndrome, Korsakoff's — síndrome de Korsakoff

syndrome, Tourette — síndrome de Gilles de la Tourette

syringe — jeringa

system — sistema

T

table — mesa

tablespoon — cuchara

tablespoonful — cucharada

tablet — tableta

tactile sensation — sensibilidad táctil

take — tomar

talk — hablar, hable

taste — saber saborear, probar [verb]; sabor [noun]

tastebud — papila gustativa

team — equipo

teaspoon — cucharita

technique — técnica, método

teeth — dientes

Teeth Sweep Exercise — ejercicio de limpiar los dientes

telephone — teléfono

telephone number — número de teléfono

temperature — temperatura

temporal — temporal

temporary — temporáneo, temporaria

tender — adolorido

tense — tenso

tension — tensión

test — prueba, examen

texture — textura

textured bolus strategy — estrategia de bolo con textura

thalamus — tálamo

therapeutic — terapéutico

therapy, speech — terapia del habla

thermal — termal

thermal stimulation — estimulación termal

Thermal-Tactile Stimulation Exercise/Strategy — ejercicio/estrategia de estimulo táctil

thick (consistency) — espeso

thicken — espesar

thickened — espesado

thin — ralo

thin liquids — líquidos ralos

think — pensar

thirsty, to be — tener sed

throat — garganta

throat, sore — dolor de garganta

thrush — infección de la boca

thyroid — tiroideo

thyroid cartilage — cartílago de tiroideo

tickle — hacer cosquillas

tight — apretado

Tight Lip Exercise — ejercicio de labio apretado

tighten — apretar

tilt — inclinar

time — tiempo

times — veces

tingle — hormiguear

tingling — hormigueo

tip — punta

tired — cansado/cansada

tissue — tejido, pañuelo

today — hoy

toe — dedo

together — junto

tolerance — tolerancia

tolerate — tolerar, aguantar

tomorrow — mañana

tone — tono

tongue — lengua

tongue — lengua

Tongue Anchor Exercise — ejercicio de anclar la lengua

tongue base — base de la lengua

Tongue Bowl Lift Exercise — ejercicio de formar un tazón y levantar la lengua

Tongue Bowl Slide Exercise — ejercicio de formar tazón y resbalar con la lengua

tongue depressor — depresor de lengua

Tongue Press Exercise — ejercicio de apretón de lengua

Tongue Squeeze Strategy — estrategia de apretón de lengua

Tongue Tickle — cosquilleo de lengua

tongue tip — la punta de la lengua

Tongue Tip Push Exercise — ejercicio de empujón de la punta de la lengua

Tongue Tip Sound Production Exercise — ejercicio de producción de sonido con la punta de la lengua

Tongue Tip Swipe Exercise — ejercicio de limpiar con la punta de la lengua

Tongue to Cheek Push Exercise — ejercicio de empujón de lengua a mejilla

tonsil — amígdala, angina

tonsillitis — amigdalitis

tooth — diente

toothbrush — cepillo de dientes

toothbrush rub — rozar del cepillo de dientes

Toothette sponge — esponjita

Toothette Sqeeze Exercise — ejercicio de apretón con esponjita

touch — tocar

towel — toalla

trace — trazas

trachea — traquea

tracheostomy — traqueostomía

train — entrenar

training — entrenamiento

transition — transición

translate — traducir

traumatic — traumático

tray — bandeja, charola

treatment — tratamiento

tremor — temblor

trial — ensayo

trigger — disparador

trouble — molestia

tube — tubo

tube, feeding — sonda para alimentación

tube, nasogastric — tubo nasogástrico

turn — vuelta

turn around — darse media vuelta

tympanic membrane — membrano timpánica

U

ulcer — ulcera

unable — incapaz

uncle — tío

uncomfortable — incomodo

unconscious — inconsciente

unresponsive — insensible

unstable — inestable

until — hasta

unusual — raro, extraño

up — arriba

upset — trastornado

upward — hacia arriba

urgent — urgente

urinate — orinar

urologist — urólogo

urosepsis — urosepsis

use — usar

usual — usual

uvula — úvula

V

vagus — vago

vallecula — valecula

Valsalva Maneuver Exercise — ejercicio de maniobra Valsalva

value — valor

variation — variación

vary — variar

Vaseline — Vaselina

velopharyngeal port — puerto velofaringeo

velum — velo del paladar

ventilate — ventilar

ventilator — ventilador

ventral — ventral

vibration — vibración

virus — virus

virus, human immunodeficiency (HIV) — virus de inmunodeficiencia humana

visit — visitar

vocal — vocal

vocal fold — cuerda vocal

vocal quality — calidad de voz

voice — voz

voluntary — voluntario/voluntaria

vomit — vomito

W

waist — cintura

wait — esperar

walker — andadera

warm — caliente, tibio

Warm Lip Rub — rozar tibio al labio

wash — lavar

Washcloth Rub — rozar con toallita

water — agua

weak — débil

wear — llevar

weigh — pesar

weight — peso

well — bien

wet — mojar

wheelchair — silla de ruedas

whichever — cualquier

while — mientras

white — blanco

wide — ancho

wife — esposa

will — voluntad

wipe — enjugar

wire — alambre

woman — mujer

work — trabajo

worse — empeorar

wrist — muñeca

X

x-ray — rayos x

x-ray film, chest — radiografia del tórax

Y

yawn — bostezar

year — años

yesterday — ayer

Z

zip code — código postal

Index

V